Autism, Pre Rain Man

Autism, Pre Rain Man

❖

Pre Rain Man Autism

Rich Shull

iUniverse, Inc.

New York Lincoln Shanghai

Autism, Pre Rain Man
Pre Rain Man Autism

iUniverse, Inc.

For information address:
iUniverse, Inc.
2021 Pine Lake Road, Suite 100
Lincoln, NE 68512
www.iuniverse.com

ISBN: 0-595-29298-4

Printed in the United States of America

To Grandma Mae

1906–1994

To Jypsy

Founder of the: The Maze, Ooops Wrong Planet web site.

A Sincere Thank you! Your Kind sincere efforts united many of the participants in this high functioning experiment together!
Perhaps, You Have the Phone the Wrong Way Around,
A Blind Backwards Experiment in Autism

Along Came Rain Man

Luella's Journey

By Rich Shull

Contents

A special thanks to the many people and friends and neighbors, teachers &tutors over the years that all blindly helped this experiment come to a successful end. A special mention to Mom, Dad, Mary Ann and Grandma. A very special thanks to Doug Buhrer who's initial editing and insight and years of support set the tone for this reading. Another very special hello to my Autistic Yahoo Groups whose friendship and support and experiences helped in this book and hopefully this, as well as, your future books will help us wake up Autism to its successful forgotten past.

1

A Personal Note From the Author

Dear Readers,

What your holding in your hand or viewing on the web is the result of nearly 40 years of blind research on Autism. I have overcome Autism as have a legion of other people worldwide and typically we drive hold normal jobs and participate in real life. It is our duty to mankind and to Autism to present this workable version of Autism on behalf of those less able to figure out their condition. Our condition as it is explained here answers lots of Autism questions and might even answer the 'missing link' question in evolution. Our odd success story and the reasons behind it are explained. Autism is easy and simple and just like "Latin". Its entire concept has never been understood by anyone in the spectrum. With that in mind I would like to bring up a point made by 19th century philosopher Authur Schopenhauer. He said, _All truth passes through three stages, one it is ridiculed, two it is violently opposed, three it is accepted as self-evident._ I suspect this reading explaining a quiet successful Autism with many unexpected truths will be ridiculed, opposed and perhaps some day seen for the obvious insight it might contain.

Thinking in Pictures The book by Temple Grandin is the closest thing to Autism perfection I have ever seen and only just grazes the tip of Autism. Even though I never met her personally Temple's work speaks for itself. I'm in sincere hopes for the sake of Autism and its people that this book takes up where Temple's book and others before it left off. Some years ago I 'seen, heard and felt' every word Temple said during her Fresh Air Radio interview and I had never heard of the word Autism: But it was clear to me my strange, odd thoughts were Picture Thoughts. I was 35 very well versed in Autism and didn't even know it. This new word Autism finally put a precise name to my condition. Prior to this I was just a strange kid. This book explains Picture Thought (Autism Thought) from baby thoughts to advanced Picture Thought the Autistics of yesterday use today. It is the same picture base thought that needs to be taught to today. It is our natural language and even our 'body language' if you know how to read it. My counterparts and I are mostly older and undiagnosed and we all learned Autism on our own and even being totally ignorant of one another we came up with the 'same' thing. For many reasons the current Autism has missed many of the points so vital to Autism. It is impossible for the traditional thinkers of this world to figure out what Autism is as it is not common thought. Thankfully it sometimes parallels normal thought or modern Autism education would never work.

Hopefully, this book will inspire everyone with in the spectrum to progress to higher standards and goals and ultimately it might lay the foundation for a school dedicated to Autism, like a deaf or blind school is today. I firmly believe there is great hope for someone Autistic and feel most Autistics would function well in society if only they were taught in their native language. Imagine spending your education experience naturally "knowing" only one language and being taught in another? Certainly, your progress would be hit and miss. Via my experiment and the similar experience of others the world over we actually in a round about way learned to think normally and Autistically. This hybrid experience might open up a lot of doors and even new medical and psychological fields. Autism in simplest terms is "thinking in French and talking in English".

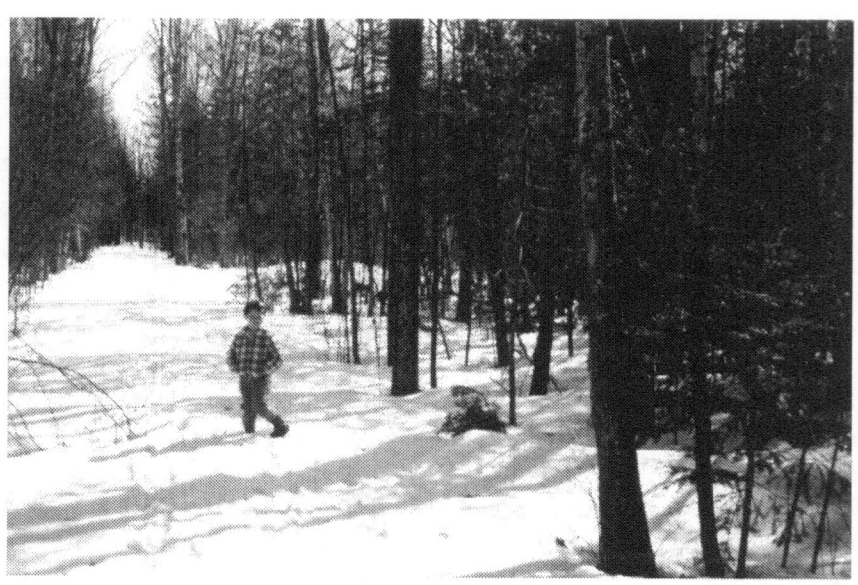

Rich, Taken in 1967(?) Larks Lake Michigan.

I have this underling fear as this goes to press that it might be too little too late. Autism these days is truly big business Political action committees, group homes and special education created in the spirit of good will. I suspect before Autism became a buzzword and a subject of semi—common knowledge after the release of the movie Rain Man Autism might have had a better chance of a more meaningful progress. Rain Man was a wonderful hit move that featured an autistic character. Sadly the results of the world seeing a good movie actually set the study of Autism back a few moments in time as lot of "facts" were presented that didn't take into account all of us that had over came Autism or our success stories, like I write about here. It seems more and more people are diagnosed Autistic in this day and age and I wonder if some are not simply behavior problems or have educational issues. Old undiagnosed Autistics like me have had to overcome and live in Rain Man's Shadow. That does its part to hide and stifle those of us on the wrong side of the timeline. I hope someday when Autism is figured out, it will be discovered there is little difference between high and low functioning autism. It is all the same stuff taught in the wrong way.

There is some advantage to going through life clueless, myself and others like me that were schooled prior to the early 70s were never diagnosed Autistic, (it wasn't possible in that era) we blundered our way through life and inadvertently taught ourselves Autism. Typically I have met my counter parts on the Internet and all of us share similar stories of blind backward development and success. Of the 160 or so I have met 30–40 of us truly are truly successful making a good salary and holding a good job, but the majority of us hold lower entry level positions since our Autistic minds work in slow motion compared to the average person. Hopefully, I can get my counterparts to write their own books like this one.

In general we are not out and about, and can be the more forgotten people of society. We might have been the odd kid in school with you or perhaps the village idiot. Thankfully, some of us have somehow created a life for ourselves but I wonder how many more of us can't be found as we do not "exist"; maybe we live in a rooming house and move often? The 'new' big business of Autism, I'm afraid will not be thrilled with this writing and will hopefully it will critique it kindly. I suspect they might not want to hear of Autism like this: it might highlight just what has been missed. We are time and answers in a bottle. When I turned to the Autism Establishment for help in writing this many years ago, I was flatly turned down. I suspect being high functioning I was not supposed to exist. There is a lot of different and perhaps bold information in this book. It ties to cover every aspect of Autistic life form Pain-Free injuries which I have had personal experience with, as well as autistic driving and social skills and even some of the "tricks of" thinking and living in the real world with an Autism based mind. We really do a normal life, we have figured out our Autism and would like to share this experience with others in the spectrum. My story and that of others like me constitutes this book and hopefully will repaint the face of Autism to something closer to what it really is.

Sincerely, Rich Shull

2

Rain Man's Curse

Long before <u>Rain Man</u> the movie, unknowingly unleashed a wild team of untamed experts to the world Autistics the world over were doing rather well on our own. Most of us before Rain Man were never diagnosed and that was indeed a blessing as there was not an expert in sight to tell us NO, we can't do that, or No, you can't teach like that or tell us or anyone associated with us not to try too hard as Autism is so dreadful and a life sentence. Well, sadly it has become just that especially in America. Just look at the Autistics in a group home after Rain Man and just try to find us in one pre Rain Man? Quite likely many of us simply out grew our Autism and perhaps made a life for ourselves via our Splinter Skills. Splinter Skills are areas of instant genius or a natural learning hallway many autistic people have. The character Rain Man was great at math and numbers, but could do little else. I am great at mechanical things and others have a gift of computers or music. Perhaps there is a more singular splinter skill such as an obsession with trains. Inadvertently, We learned most of our life skills via our splinter skills, no one was there to tell our tutors and teachers splinter skills were a' horrible idea'.

Many of us are not all that successful in real life in the terms of living a perfect life with home cars and families and money to spend but we are living on our own. Perhaps we live in a rooming house, and get our health care (United States) at a fee clinic or the health department? Just what highly paid researcher would dream of looking for us in those "dirty locations". If they did they would find Picture Thinkers that don't know how special they are, and perhaps even at the age of 30–40 or above have never heard of the word Autism? But they know the effects of it perfectly well. Autism is a one sided/lop sided brand of Latin that is every bit as good as normal thought but simply not a natural language for most of the population as it is for us. Autism is not mental retardation or developmental disability It is just Latin. In fact if it were taught correctly it could be as simple as a 6-year pre school, where the student could then be mainstreamed. Even the worst among us could be "well off" if taught in our native language. Many of us world-wide have already done this 6-year Latin experiment and with a little insight it could be applied to modern Autism.

You would not dream of sending your kid Autistic or otherwise to a school that was totally unqualified to teach. But yet, that is exactly what happens in Autism. In addition to the numberline and alphabet over the chalkboard the Autisc class-room would need a picture chart to tell us about or thoughts, Yes WE have dif-ferent thoughts than you and they might be represented like the chalkboard numberline. For the first time ever the Autistic thought from the baby thoughts upward would be recognized! Putting it another way how would you expect your kid to learn "Spanish" in 12 years of school if you taught him in "English" and "French"? It wouldn't work well and might just resemble modern Autism, after Rain Man.

Thanks to the Internet Service Yahoo perhaps 70–80 of high functioning Autistic people actively participate in Autism real life. Most of us do what Autism claims as impossible we hold normal jobs, drive and have families. Most of us have Pic-ture Thought figured out and have successfully worked it into real life. We often talk of how and what type of Picture thought we use, how to convert that normal thought and how we blend our wild senses into everyday life. We even clue in newer younger members of our group that were diagnosed autistic in school as to their Picture Thought and watch them blossom. It is amazing just what can hap-pen even late in life if the natural proper language is taught. Most of us made it by accident and figured out despite the fact no one else in the world knew that we had 'funny' picture thought' as well as 'normal thought'. Working hard in school and NOT knowing of Autism made that success possible. No one told us we were dumb Autistic or otherwise and as such we learned to try and try and try again and others like our teachers and tutors all joined in our fight and it worked. Many of us learned most of our stuff via accident via splinter skills. Once you understand Autism you will see the perfect reasoning to this currently UNAP-PROVED learning method. Our Splinter skills made us appear smart to the untrained onlooker and soon by 8th grade most of us learned (unknowingly) enough of autism to function on our own. Some of us still fooled everyone by being on the honor roll on time and being considered for Special Education the next time report cards were issued.

In real life we have figured out little tricks and secrets to deal with the traditional thinkers and sadly have also discovered entire new aspects of medicine. We are painless when it comes to injuries, many of us have walked away from car accidents and worse "unhurt" just to go to the Emergency Room days and weeks and perhaps months later as we just now felt the injuries or more likely the effects of them. Walk into the ER a day late and a dollar short, not feeling any pain and just see if anyone believes you? Then the ER Staff calls the Autism Society of America or goes to their website or someone else's to discover all kinds of diets and perhaps a small blurb that some kids show little reaction to pain? When X-rays are finally done the entire ER goes "Dead quiet" and the staff and doctors gather around the viewing light and GASP he really is hurt! He was telling the Truth! I probed him so hard and he felt nothing, didn't even wince! These are some of the comments you hear, as well as the worst one, I was never taught anything about this in Medical school!

Perhaps the oldest Autistic person I know if she were still living (2003) would be 70 some years old now and was the first Autistic I ever met. I had just been diagnosed after reading Temple's book and also just suffered a serious injury that I knew I had but it seemed impossible for anyone to detect. "Fay" was on an internet board with a listing of ODD Medicine and that is where we met. She told me of the lumps and tumors she had associated with female type trouble. She never felt any of that stuff! But her doctors did and after surgery learned the doctors were horrified of the actual size of that stuff and the idea she never felt it? She to thought in Pictures and learned it on her own and commented to me Rain Man dashed all hopes of ever figuring out the Autism the world really should know. She thought it would nearly impossible to fight Hollywood and now a boatload of questionable 'experts' looking for a free un-critqued career researching autism. "Who cares if more autistic kids end up in a group home, as long as a doctors Malibu home is paid for?" from Fay.

Thankfully the next place I found on the net was Jupsy's Other Planet Website. Jupsy's web site is a BIG list of all kinds of Autism resources. It literally got me in contact with the right people and it saved my life gave me some bearing and sanity. My (our) Hat is off to the wonderful service Jupsy has done for the world of Autism. SHE IS THE SAINT OF AUTISM. As of this writing her advanced stages of Multiple Sercious are taking their toll on her life and it is reported she is having a harder and harder time keeping up with life. She has done plenty so far! Thanks again for saving and helping so many people!

Really Autistic?

In my many years of autism and since being officially diagnosed 9 years ago now I have met many people from all over the Autism spectrum. I do wonder if some of them are not Autistic? There is an Epidemic after all, perhaps of fiscal nature? I have seen where football star Doug Fluite's son is "cured" of autism? Well that is great news if it is true but even the best of the old "war horses' among us that function really well and yes, even drive have also "cured autism" but our wild senses and Autism's other permanent quirks never go away they are just hidden.

I have set along side many "autistic" at a MAAP (More Able Autistic People) conference in Indiana USA in a room set aside for Autistics to 'get away' only to be treated to a visible display of Autism Vs Non Autistic? Pots and pans being dropped in a hall way perhaps close to a kitchen startled everyone autistic in the room as this is a natural occurrence for us as we hear so much more than the Traditional Thinker does. Some in the room were totally UN phased with the noise. Just like Mom and Dad and our teachers and doctors are not effected by it.

I can't help but wonder if a lot of modern Autism is just simply behavior trouble, and then if you treat the kid Autistic—suddenly—he becomes Autistic? In my day before Rain Man many of us had our behavior trouble to and even a number of us were dyslexic and even had ADD but I dare say a strict upbringing while painful for the parents cured us of those troubles. I even over come Encholoia the Autistic trait of having to say a word no matter what, and learned to hold the word until I was out of hearing range of Mom or Dad. Anything I said would have been considered "Talking Back", an absolute 'no-no'. That has really helped socially today as I learned just to hold the word (hard to do) and say it later when I will not look like a fool. Even in my day kids were paddled and if you got one at school you also got one at home to, even the bus drivers could paddle their passengers! Paddling is not Child abuse, so don't get your knickers in a twist, and in most cases it was the last resort punishment. It seems more like behavior modification. Granted some folks DID take advantage of it and turn it into child abuse. I know if Dad would have known of the autistic Pain Tolerance he would have taken that into consideration before the punishment was administered and I was never abused anyway. In general most of the older Autistics I have met all credit those early learned lessons in life with some of their success of today.

Old Autistics often tell of the coming of age of fluorescent lights a big event in public buildings in starting in the 1940's they drove us crazy. It seems Autistics could see the cycle change (room got brighter and darker in a constant fashion) in the room on dark days or all the time if it was in interior room. I even experienced some of those lights as late as the mid 1990's at the Nosinger Center on the Ohio State University Campus. Starting in the 1970's most of the older lights were replaced or the parts converted to phase the light and the cycle change is no longer visible to us. That might be a good test for Autism?

Of Course, hearing is another form of "Autistic Latin" and one our normal thinking 'experts' are ignorant of. If they can't hear it how can we hear it? It could be done but we need a test to look for super good hearing well above the range of the typical person. We can tell you what noise caused every dog in the neighborhood to start barking (usually a distant siren) and all the high pitches and screams of Mom's voice stuff she is unaware of, we know when the kid down the street is practicing the flute.

As for Pain Tolerance that seems to be an Autistic trait that might be tested for by having someone tighten a series of bolts until they are tight. The autistic person would probably break the bolts thinking they were not tight. If some one were not autistic it seems they might actually tighten the bolt and not break it. When I (we) meet our counter parts many don't have any trouble with noise, vision (being real sensitive) or pain tolerance and none seem to Think in Pictures or have a clue to what were talking about. Even some younger folks that suffered through brainwashing report realizing their picture thought if we explain it to them. I guess it is possible to be Autistic and not picture think but I would expect most to realize instantly their odd thought process. For the non-picture thinkers I would expect (and sometimes get) an odd explanation of their thoughts that for sure are not normal thought. I can see where some Autistics especially modern ones might never have had the chances we had to develop their picture thought but, it would seem they still have the basic thought, just not in visual form.

A mix of real Autistic people and presumed Autistic people muddy the waters and skew the many studies of Autism short changing both sides. A Non-autistic autistic might respond well to hugs, personal attention and feel pain in a typical sense, where as a true Autistic would not enjoy a hug, true personal attention and definitely does NOT feel a lot of pain. If by chance there are a lot of UN Autistic Autistics in the mix Autism needs to weed out the mix and do what is best for both parties. Perhaps, true Autistics might actually get better more to the point care.

Education, Two Steps Backward, & a "Worthless" Benchmark Book.

Didn't anyone comprehend Temple's wonderful book <u>Thinking in Pictures?</u> It seems lots of people have read her book but few if any applied the information in it to real autistic life. Really a SING-A-LONG for Autistic Kids? Simply get a gun out and shoot your self in the foot, it is has the same effect. Basically Autistics can only really use one sense at a time really effectively (especially during learning) and the senses we do have like hearing are far more precise and beyond the range of your hearing that experience. Doing too much with the senses at one time causes overload. Sitting in that sing-a-long would be an Autistic nightmare. No it might not hurt us physically, but we would for sure not function the entire time were setting there being force fed the "best" of education. The small little overloads that would spark would in effect leave us "dead" 85% of the time were participating in the group.

Even in the best of times us older Autistics have a time handling two or three things at once. Many of us experience our BEST Autistic to Normal person communication via the telephone. If were in a QUIET room and there is a clear connection we can talk and *read our picture thoughts and convert them to speech to be spoken.* That indeed takes lots of brainpower to do that. So now add to the mix people walking into the room, the screech of mom's voice (that normal people don't hear) or worse yet the television blaring away in that room or even a distant one and we no longer can hear the other person talk to us easily. It also interferes with our picture processing and speech conversion, and indeed were true experts at it and know and understand our Picture Thought. If that type of behavior ruins us, just think of trouble it is causing an Autistic person in a sing-a-long, one perhaps that doesn't even have a clue to the picture thought process. If young Autistics had a clue to their native language, all would protest that type of learning environment as they instantly realize their thoughts are being stifled with all that processing that could not be done easily. As it is our native thought is the "Spanish" that is never being taught to us and even brainwashed from us in the disguise of helping? Many of us older undiagnosed Autistics will tell you most of our quality learning happened alone in a quieter place like at a tutors home, or at our own home in a quiet house, perhaps even out of doors if we lived in the country. School in general had to be library quiet (no echo's please) for maximum learning.

Even today a quiet house is a loud house when, we came home from school there was typically no TV to watch or Video's to play or music to download and thus the house was quiet, perfect for homework, or just Autistically relaxing and catching up with our thoughts. I bet the modern Autistic is "never there" or processing but precious little of the information being presented to him or her. Of course, Normal kids with out a thought conversion process probably take in lots more of the stuff presented to them. When were in overload the lights are on but no one is home to make matters worse we learn to look (by Accident) respond to key things in our environment "just in time" so that we look like were more connected than we are. In fact I bet the autistic kid may not realize or have heard the instructions of the teacher to 'get up' move etc. but simply followed along with the action of the others.

The good news is older Autistics in the real world are a bit social and participate in the lives of others and our partners, families and co-workers, The only reason we really do that well is we have figured out our natural thought process and the world we live in and in so many words cured Autism. But putting a kid in a sing-a-long with out the entire Autism process not in prospective is worthless. Many of us in the real world use hearing filters, pre think our possible conversations, and even use "sign language" in bars and pubs.

Temple's entire book at times seems to be ignored; even her ideas on splinter skill learning are ignored. I don't think it is anything personal with her quality work it is rather the audience reading it. EVERYTHING she says although true goes against the grain of what a traditional thinker is expecting to hear or can relate to and as such is falsely interpreted in to normal thought. Perhaps she has never been given the chance to really express her thoughts at a speaking engagement. Traditional Thinkers are likely to put words in her mouth they want to hear and relate to. It seems modern people don't have the time to wait for our complete correct answer, and those of in the real world make provisions for that.

Autism's Hope

If we might turn back time and remove the hype from Autism and possibly turn it into a the unknown condition it might have been before Rain Man I suspect there would not be an epidemic of cases and instead of diets galore better research might have yield by now the idea we really have a different thought process. Perhaps it might realize that we turn our Optic nerves off and on and one moment see what you see and the next are thinking with a brain generated image (picture thought). Those of us that really do the real world would be sought after for our information and insight. Currently for sometime now we have been vigorously ignored by The Autism Establishment that just can not admit to us, think of the "egg on their face" if we were admitted to? All of those poor folks in a group home don't have to be there? Think of the "Diet Doctors" their careers are at stake? Perhaps the lawsuits might switch from vaccines to the advice given since Rain Man?

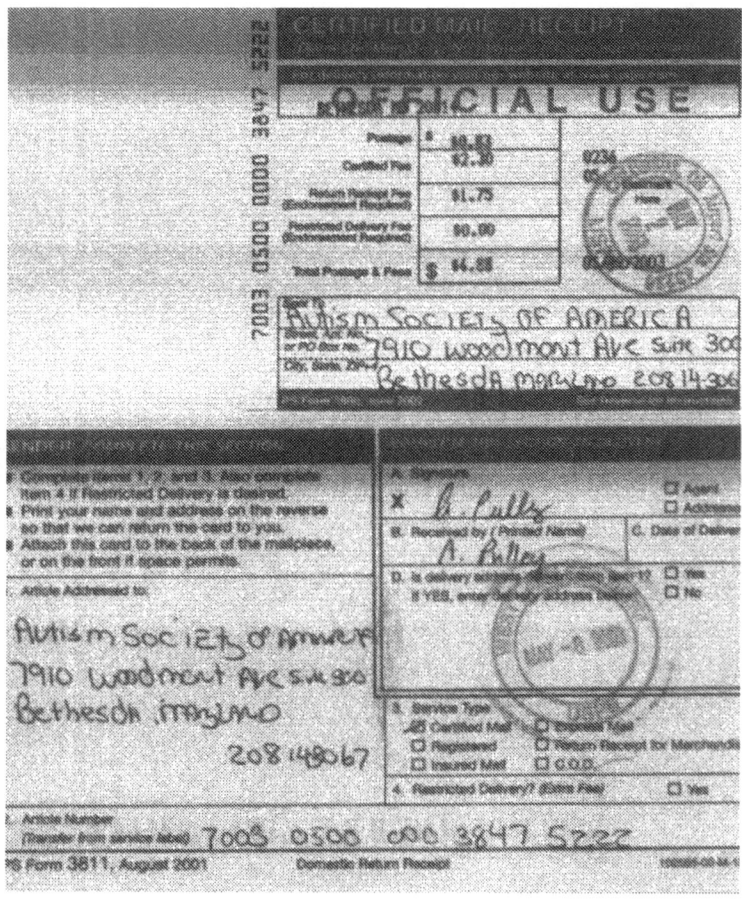

Pictured above are receipts of certified mail asking to be represented at the Autism Society of Americas July 2003 Conference in Pittsburgh Pa. USA.

Some7–8 years ago now I sent the first edition of this book to the Autism Society of America and Dr Rimland and another, autism research non profit and never heard one thing from anyone of them. Since then my quest has expanded and includes my High-functioning counterparts worldwide. The above registered mail receipts show this years (2003) attempt at is recognized at the ASA Convention. As you can read the mail was received but I was never personally contacted or were my follow-up emails returned. Plus I spent hours on hold with the ASA and never spoke to a person. I did find the website of an ASA board member who informed me if I paid the full price there were several open forums where one could speak. I bet my speakers slip would remain on the bottom of that list forever? If they ignore you for 7 years, talking in person on a subject they don't want to know about seems like Autism's impossible dream.

A friend of mine that suffers from the worst form of pain known to man called Cluster Headaches often comments at least Rain Man was not about this or we might be researched to death by now like Autism is. We often joke of the 'cluster-head diet" that hasn't been invented yet. Clusterheads often take Rx Morphine to control their pain and a good day is hard to come by. We often comment that we will know when the science of medicine has finally done something when they discover the cure for the clusterheads and the pain free life of an Autistic person. Not so Ironically there is precious little research being done on cluster headaches as one there isn't many people afflicted with them and there is little chance of fame and fortune and perhaps most important there is not a network of non-profits set up to 'help". That prevents lots of media spin and might even keep some less than sincere professionals from entering the field. In fact a lot of their limited research comes from doctors that are also afflicted. Curing both of these conditions at each end of the pain spectrum might go light years in helping mankind in general.

Our Autism Answers

Between my self and my counterparts and friends worldwide, we constitute Autism's last hope. We are Autism's last undiagnosed populations that blindly overcame our condition. We know Autism is not a simple subject but yet so many of us do what is claimed as impossible. Were on to something like it or not. In fact we propose setting up an Autism school, the first one ever that would actually teach Autism in the correct environment. We are sure to have many advantages over anyone else attempting to figure out autism as we have already been there figured it out and participated in the real world. What traditional thinking expert can make that claim? They haven't even had a Picture Thought! (Obviously!)

The study of Autism shouldn't worry to much about our success in educating our selves as we will open four times as many doors as we close when our successful students graduate school. We have entire different brains and thought than normal people, our senses could be studied for years on end. Our thought process, figured out might actually solve all kinds of other trouble like mental illness and explain lot of learning disabilities. Granted the not so stellar Doctors might lose out on an easy career but, I shouldn't worry about them too much, they might jump ship and research something else. I would not expect them to leave during telethon season however.

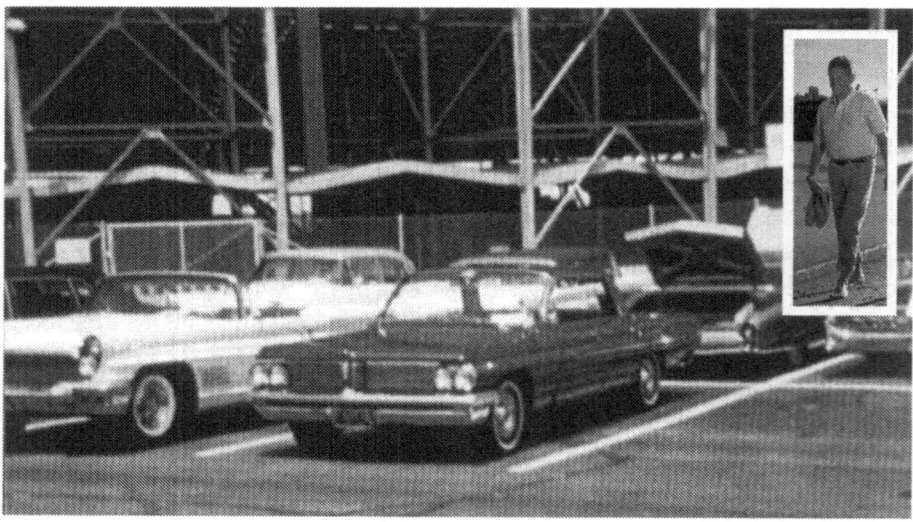

The above Picture is an advanced Autistic thought, It requires the knowledge of still pictures, motion pictures like those mentioned in <u>Thinking in Pictures</u>, as well as, many more type of pictures (thoughts). As odd as this thought appears to a normal thinker it can be rather common for an Autistic person. Typically the older we are (not diagnosed) the more we use complicated pictures of this nature to think and communicate with. We know of NO Autism Expert that has ever had a thought like this, besides those of us naturally programmed Autistic. Of Course, that either means 'were off our rockers' or dead right. I sure there will be experts of all types chiming in from all points of view. We welcome their comments and would really appreciate it IF they sit down and listen to our story.

As for the picture above the little picture in the corner, might be like a daydream a normal thinker would experience. In our case that picture tell us all kinds of stuff, sometimes that picture in the corner fills in our entire visual field and we no longer see the Red Car, but yet you would still see it if we were standing beside each other. Of Course you never see our thought picture in the corner. That is a brain-generated image we use to think with. I think we use our optic nerve and brain in conjunction to make our Autism thoughts work. Your Autistic kids might have pictures like this, or probably less complicated thought or maybe even "blank thoughts" and by accident they are totally ignored Us older folks also ignored them growing up until we discovered by accident just how useful they were. Why didn't other students or the teacher mention these types of thoughts? Traditional Thinkers don't have clue to this type of thought and if we mention the pictures and talk of them too often were asking for a trip to the funny farm. Of course, as many of us that made it know, or figured out eventually that we do have a different thought process than normal and it is best not to bother others with it.

Before you discount Autistic thought yet again, and get out the brainwashing manuals take a moment to realize it Fathered the Computer via the talents of a man by the name of Dr Alan Turing (1912–1954). Lots of smart people the world over have been claimed to be Autistic or have Autistic traits. For sure our naturally different point of view assures you and us that we will be the ones to really come up with the different ideas. We indeed have so many experts in our high functioning group in many different professions. Yours truly has invented a new internal combustion motor that promises to be 70% efficient. I have also devised ways to make Auto Repair fool proof by combining my experience and knowledge of cars along with my ultra senses to invent new machines to help diagnose and fix things. With a little luck parts replacement as diagnosis will be a thing of the past, even if the Model T motors we are still using are really primitive.

Please, read the book carefully and realize it is the author's personal experience. But, also remember there are many others like me with similar stories to tell. Despite the fact we were all ignorant of one another and mostly in different parts of the world we all have developed similar versions of Autism Thought. It seems we all started with the same types of thought and moved on to the next step naturally progressing up the Autism Thought scale, just like kids learn to read a t the 3 grade level or 5 Th. grade level. We all seemed to learn how to control our Thought Pictures so that we can blend together normal thought like you use so we can participate in life and do things like drive. We all have a special twist to our thought probably since we all learned Autism on our own. Some of us have and use 3 and 4-d thoughts and some combine sound with the thoughts and yet others seem to have a sound based Autism thought process. All of this constitutes Autism and the answers to its many mysteries. Our experiences and a school based on them (ran by us initially) will bring autism out of the dark ages and hopefully mend some mistakes of the past and even create a my dream Autism learning program—A 6 year Autism/Latin pre school.

3

The Pictures of Autism

It seems one the most important parts of Autism, the pictures, are seemingly the only thing dealing with Autism that are not talked about by anyone within the Autism spectrum. That's hardly a surprise, many Autistics themselves don't realize what their pictures are. Plus the pictures are "invisible concepts" to anyone else. Out of sight out of mind as the old adage goes. I predict the psychological establishment will be lost and doubtful with this explanation but the real key to understanding Autism is mastering the thought pictures. Once understood the real difference between the normal thinker and the Autistic thinker will point out why we are so different. The communication impasse, the lack of empathy, and the Autistic's need for reason in decision making and the poor outcomes of things might finally be grasped. Please keep the picture explanations your about to read in mind through the book. Autistic thoughts develop, naturally but no one knows what to do with it. The Autistic person sees them develop in his mind (what are those?) No one else even makes a mention of them in school or at home and suddenly his best chance at understanding his/her natural programmed language is ignored. It is assumed, although they call us Autistic we think normally as that 'normal thought' is what they try teach us and then we get some MR/DD labels when we don't meet their 'normal standards'. Autism is simply thinking in one language and talking in another. In Fact you might think of this book as a foreign language course, that teaches an internal and external version of Autism.

Thanks to <u>Thinking in Pictures</u> the pictures we think with and work with, were brought out of the closet. The non-Autistic's daydream might be similar in concept, except Autistics literally see these thoughts. We use your "daydreams" to think with. I now understand these thoughts are not common to everyone and it only took me 34 years to figure it out. I spent the last few years with dad trying to understand his thought process. Dad is logically the one to compare thoughts with, as we understood each other before the Autism discovery. Although he really didn't totally understand me we had developed a special understanding of one another. The difference is striking, and we still have lots to learn from one another.

My styles of thought pictures, which may be shared by other autistics, are divided into several categories: **Still pictures, motion pictures and picture-in-picture** thoughts. A typical thought may only be one style, or a combination of the three. Any of these thoughts, thought-pictures can be enlarged to the point where they block the actual image being received by my eyes. The Deeper or "fuller "the thought, the greater the chance the optic image may be blocked. Tony Langdon my autistic counterpart in Australia has even more complicated thoughts than I do at times: there 4-deminsion.

All pictures regardless of style are "real" as those viewed with my eyes. Color detail and prospective are accurate. My pictures are never in black and white. Sleep dreams are not conscious, but my pictures are. Oddly, my sleep dreams seem so beautiful and carefree and are usually in no way related to my picture thoughts. I can control my pictures, and they relate to the reality of the moment, as it unfolds around me.

Perhaps, another explanation for the non-autistic is to imagine a sleeping dream, experienced while you're awake and fully conscious. You know, from having been suddenly awakened while dreaming the dreams seem incredibly real while they are happening. The fact that the dreams are often fantastic doesn't always impress as much as the feeling that what you experienced seemed "real". When you awake, you may want to share, by describing, this intense experience in words. Still you wish there were a way to communicate this fantastic experience with others. This is much like the autistic thought process, some of the best thoughts an autistic has are often "locked-in" his mind as the means to communicate and in our case translate the thought isn't developed. There will be more on picture translation later in the book.

Still Pictures

Still pictures were the first pictures I remember. It's possible I experienced these as far back as first grade, but my earliest complete memory of a still picture is from fourth grade. A homework reading assignment in social studies described the changing seasons. The lesion was accompanied by an illustration of a tree changing colors in the fall. The next day, the picture of the tree appeared in my mind in the form of an odd "post card picture" long before the class again studied the book as a whole. Later, the teacher began discussing the book and the picture appeared again. Finally, the whole class looked at the illustration in the book, confirming the accuracy of my earlier pictures. This left me puzzled, and gave me the sensation of having some form of extra sensory perception. Of course, If I had known that this type of picture was normal for Autistics and that I was the only one in the class to "see" it, I'd felt greatly relieved. As it was I tried my best to ignore these pictures from that moment on through most of eighth grade, and thought of them as a nuisance.

These pictures must be similar to a key thought a normal thinker has. These thoughts directly relate to whatever thought I need to create or possibly a thought I need to look at again. For example, my first thought and acquaintance with the Peanuts comic strip was when mom brought me the book *A Charlie Brown Christmas* by Charles Schultz. That book cover features Snoopy laughing, Charlie Brown holding a small twig of a Christmas tree and Lucy and Violet pointing, created my first thought of Charlie Brown. After reading the book, which was mostly pictures, it became basis for a lot of social development as well. Since Autistics relate to pictures naturally little did mom know this book was to become my bible. I learned a lot of social behavior based on that reading and used it well into high school as an etiquette book of all things. I'm sure the late Charles Schultz never intended it to be enjoyed in that manner.

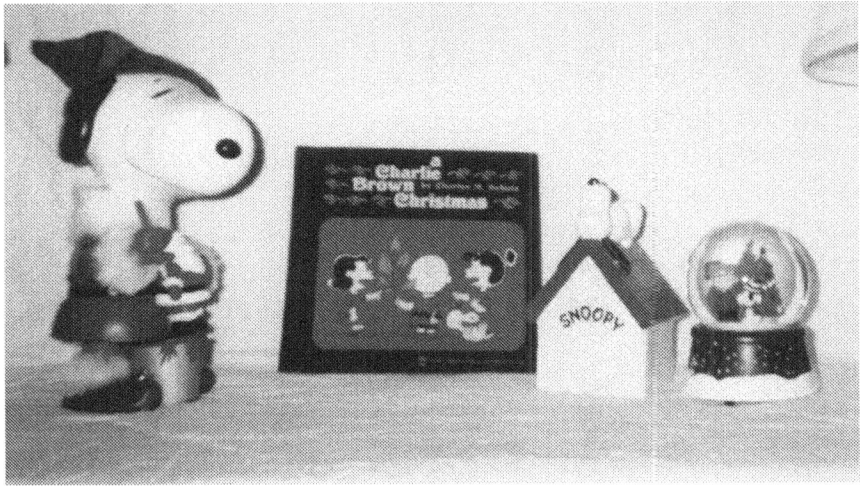

The book A Charlie Brown Christmas, my first Autism textbook.

Initially after I received the book I pretty much ignored it but soon I found my self-looking at it almost all the time. Whenever the pushy girl in our class needed to make her point on something I always found my self-looking at a picture of Lucy in the blue dress screaming something. Whenever the pushy classmate was put in her place I had a picture of Lucy being licked by Snoopy. As you might expect I could always relate to Charlie Brown, the respected oddball. The pictures I'm referring to are both my picture thought and the also the book in general, initially I used a combination of both the books real pictures and my thought pictures when I referenced something to the book.

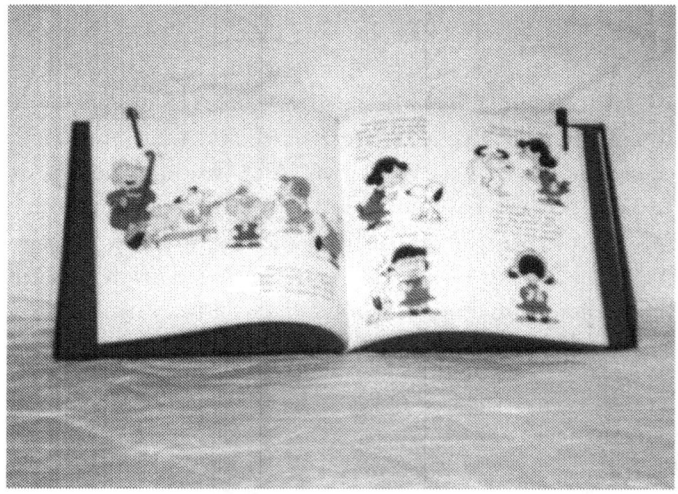

Lucy and Snoopy, one of the highlighted learning experiences.

After school I found my self going to that book time and again, I'd look at specific picture that related to what had happened at school, and then I combined several of the pictures not intended to be together by folding the pages and viewing a newly created page from opposite pages, which end in the end gave me the ideas for a new thought or solution to a problem. This was training for the picture thoughts I use today.

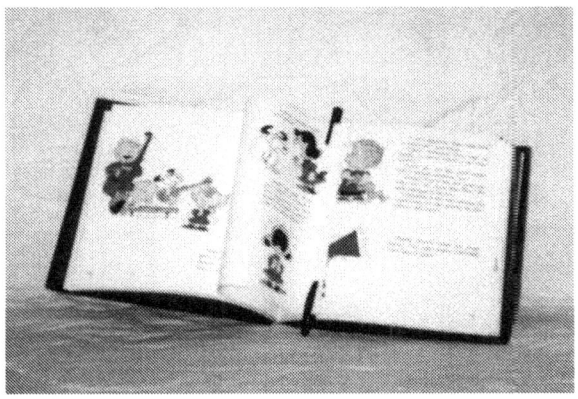

Example of new thought from folded pages.

Picture thoughts weather there the cartoon characters type thoughts like these early first pictures or the more reality based ones of today are still common thoughts. Yes, I do have a photographic memory to a large degree, but the Autistic process takes them a step or two beyond just a picture. If we were looking at the same picture and both knew all of the circumstances of the picture, you would look at the picture and say, "that's Grandpa." I on the other had would analyze that picture to the point of no return, it would spur other picture thoughts for me that might include a mental picture of his house, a picture of his mail box (showing me the address) thoughts (pictures) of his wife and kids and even a quick non picture related "smell" of his house. This wild process will tell me stuff you knew instantly, where he was from etc. Over time I learned by observation what it was you were getting out of that picture and tailored my thoughts to match.

As you can guess keeping those picture thoughts in order is a task that kept getting bigger and bigger as I experienced new things. Almost every event added a new set of thought (picture) to my memory banks. Out of necessity I finally developed out of necessity an A/B/C filing system to aid in cataloging those thoughts (pictures). Not surprisingly the system has filtered into my life at large. How many of you have a garage in alphabetical order? I can find anything in an instant, ask my neighbors.

Those 26 alphabetical "still picture markers" (thoughts) I use would be closely described as flash cards. Usually the markers consist of the flash card "picture thought" letter I need to see and from there I relate it to my alphabetical workshop or to my thoughts, in which some are in a-b-c order. For Example if I want to find my dry wall screws, I first see the letter "D", in the form of a Flash card, picture thought, from there I see the "d" crate in my work shop and usually the picture I see in my mind is 100% correct, and shows me what is in the box and how its laid out. It is wrong occasionally especially if dad has returned something to the box since I'd last seen it. Obviously it is a waste of brain power to look at a picture of a box and its contents so I try to just Think "D" and not study "D". While I'm studying the content of the "D" box and the detail of it, I could be missing the important thoughts someone is trying to communicate to me, so I now try to avoid the details of any thought, unless it is really needed. This has really sped up my communication.

Still pictures are especially useful when I need data about an object. My mind enlarges and creates a full-size image of the object I wish to study. Then, much like a laser—light pointer, I focus my "sight" to where I need additional information, say to measure the length or angle of the object. Via another special version of the still picture I can "see" the stretch of a bolt as it is torqued (tightened) or the imperfect union of two parts, or the current flowing through an electrical circuit. Just like todays computer graphics used in engineering and advertising stimulates and helps your mind explain the concept of something, this type of picture is a common mental thought process for me. It's too bad my communication skills didn't yet match my picture ability I had stuff figured out long before I could communicate it. Obviously, emotions somewhat of a learned process for an Autistic had yet to be enhanced at this point.

Motion pictures are my most useful of my mental pictures. They can be full-sized or in the picture-in-picture format. These pictures completely involve my attention so I try to avoid walking or driving, or other activities that require my conscious mind. To do otherwise it risks causing an accident. To avoid motion pictures in general I simply don't think about a subject too deeply. I suspect only 30% of my thought might be normal without pictures.

In particular, history questions or subjects almost guarantee the start of a motion picture. The pictures drift back in time, hold for partial translation, start again for additional information, hold again for another partial translation, and then the thought can be compiled for a verbal answer. The normal thinker again simply recites an answer with ease.

Motion pictures as described in <u>Thinking in Pictures</u>, can be compared to operating a VCR on fast forward or rewind. Future events can be predicted using motion pictures. For example, while driving I'm able to measure the speed and the action of other drivers and their possible moves and reactions with a 'lite' form of my motion pictures.

My first motion picture is unforgettable. Our 8th grade science teacher had just finished a lecture on combustion and had made the statement light is not a necessary product of combustion, as you can't see inside a cylinder (of an engine) anyway. I wanted to respond it was necessary, for I was "seeing" the combustion inside of an engine. My viewpoint was as if I was setting on the edge of a piston, riding it up and down, and watching the valves open and close. Even the details were complete: the type of metal used in the engine, and the poor combustion of this particular engine in my picture. Here I was riding the "computer animation" a Chevrolet Vega motor having the ride of my life (1976) hanging on to the piston.

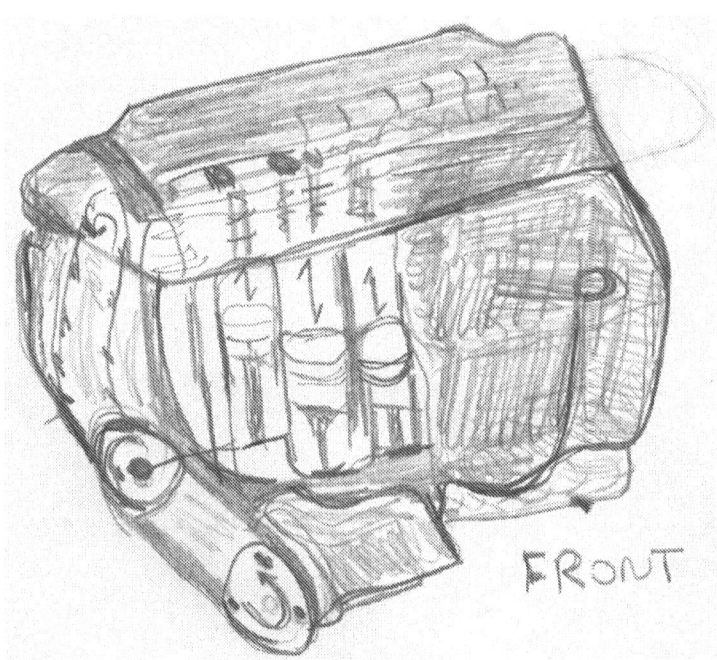

This is a similar picture to the real picture thought I had experienced in eighth grade, Now imagine it in motion, like a cartoon, and then think of it as a technical training film, possibly on how a motor works!

The wealth of information I gained or realized from that experience could have filled a 25-page report had I been able to communicate the findings. The report if it could have been written would have included the physics and the geometry and even the chemistry of the combustion event. Not surprising my mechanical splinter skills played a large roll in this massive spurt of development, coupled with today's communication ability I might have been the Enstein of the Science class. I wonder if I had already known the stuff I discovered but simply the comment made by the teacher spurred the all the right events to make for the motion picture. Years later I had a real life similar picture experience, that actually worked, when I designed the new brake system for my car using the similar pictures.

Fortunately, I contained my joy and refrained from making any statement. My reputation for being strange didn't grow stronger: at least not on that day. From then on I started paying attention to all my pictures. This motion picture was as puzzling in some respects as the 1st. Still picture was in fourth grade. If I had known of Picture Thought and what it meant to my thought process I'm sure I'd had my 1st. Motion picture years before in 5th or 6th grade. After the motion picture I somehow realized those pictures really did mean something.

Through out high school I never had any really organized thoughts, I often seen pictures during lectures mostly still pictures and many times my "social index" was linked to the Charlie Brown book (hardly the social standard for a high school student). In fact it was after I got home from school when it was quiet enough to think that I often developed pictures around what had happened at school. Sometime I put several pictures together and formed solutions to problems. It was late in college that I put all my thoughts in A-B-C order and the motion pictures really exactly matched the reality of the moment.

Picture-in-picture is a late development and combines still pictures with motion pictures and the optic picture we all see. It is exactly the same concept as a picture-in-pictue television set, where the main program your watching fills the large screen, and the smaller box within the screen holds a secondary program. For me this means my optic vision fills the large screen, and my thoughts fill the smaller screen in the corner. (Upper right generally)

As an example, the thought "Where is my Coat?" would show the large screen, filled with whatever I happened to be looking at the moment. (the same thing you would see) meanwhile, the smaller thought screen. Or window would show the coat hanging on its peg in the stairway. If I decide to retrieve my coat, I've learned it's better to focus on the vision screen. Were I to attempt to focus on the thought picture at the same time, I would be more likely to trip or walk into a piece of furniture. Picture-in-picture thought if you will is my common thought. The little pictures in the corner of my visual field give me the ability to think "gracefully" as long as, the thoughts are not too complicated. More serious thoughts require full sized pictures.

When a picture-in-pictue thought becomes "full sized" it simply enlarges to replace the optic reception. Just as you would press a button on your remote control to turn on or off the picture-in picture feature of a television set, my picture-in–picture thoughts simply appear in the corner of my optic vision. Maybe I have an automatic "Button Presser" hard wired in my thoughts. It would seem to be one of the few automatic thought processes. Still pictures and motion pictures follow suit and simply fade in and out of my thoughts. Obviously, mind imposed pictures filling up my optical field are somewhat dangerous especially while walking or driving. In fact I might be looking right at you and not see you at all; at times my optic nerve is being shorted by the brain allowing me to think about the subject at hand with a picture (thought). This is why we miss the social clues in fact, you might be sticking out your tongue at me while were talking and I'd probably miss it!

Now that we have some idea of the pictures that is only half of the thought concept, they have to be translated into understandable speech relevant to the conversation at hand. One does not realize just how fast normal conversation flows until it needs to be Autistically processed. The picture processing is easy compared to this: probably because the pictures are natural, for us, just like normal thought is for you. This is the point where a translator between say someone deaf and someone hearing might take place. Only no one can see our pictures thus we have to rely on ourselves to translate them.

Development of these thought pictures was a gradual and trail and error process. They were an automatic process to a large degree" natural" if you will. I now realize they were in a developing stage from my kindergarten days on. Usually they were small glimpses of something, a flash of a "black dot', in the same position where my picture-in-picture thoughts appear today. In Fact I often wondered why I had seen all of those spots? Sadly they were also automatically ignored, I never heard the teacher or my other classmates mention look at your thought picture regarding so and so.

These undeveloped and unrealized picture thoughts if somehow been allowed to develop naturally assure me I'd been thinking in Pictures well before 8th grade. The general development was really puzzling and often shocking when I realized the pictures and my "normal" thoughts related to the reality of the moment. Even more amazing everything I learned was tied into a picture thought. I'm still at a loss figuring if my picture thoughts are a de-fault thought process, mother natures, last attempt to get a human to think or it could be a super advanced thought process as well but that doesn't stand to reason either as if it were our senses would be probably be more normal. I also wonder if an Autistic thinks more like a dog might think?

To re-cap, still thoughts (pictures) seem to develop naturally and probably appear in the pre school time of life. Motion pictures follow and possibly even start around fourth grade. Finally if one has some normal thought ability I would guess Picture-in-picture thought would develop from there. Of Course, none of this picture development let alone how to deal with it is even considered in the current education system. Obviously, a lot of educational progress made by an Autistic is probably by chance and made only by those blindly figuring out some difference in their thought and normal thought. If an Autism School similar to a Deaf School could be Established I'd predict 70% of Autistics simply realizing their differences and re-channeling their efforts could learn how to relate to normal society and have little trouble living a normal life. As I see it once the conversion process is made form one type of thought to another, like an interface on a computer someone Autistic could handle life better.

Translating pictures to "English": Noise as a factor

Now that we realize the possible type of pictures, drop any ideas that they're like the pictures contained in your photo album. Instead convert all the pictures in you album to an engineering drawing, and cartoons include stupid details like a materials list and demensions. Of course, my mechanical nature might preclude that I naturally translate my pictures in to something similar to an engineering drawing, someone musical might have a different point of view. Never the less, I suspect the Autistic might get something totally different out of whatever picture s/he is looking at.

The Autistic has great difficulty in relating his or her pictures to others. Not only is the level of detail hard to describe, remember when I said I thought my first motion picture would be worth a 25-page report? We mistakenly assume the non-autistic think likes us, we have no other point of view to relate to. The same can be said for the normal thinker he hasn't clue to what "normal" for an autistic thinker might be. Almost every word to can be the equivalent to a chapter in a book for the non-autistic. I'll bet some of my "key "words can have 30 or 40 pictures associated with them, some times all the versions need sorted out, if the thought is developing badly. Probably this due to the fact it's more complicated than the average thought, in most circumstances only a few key pictures are necessary to figure out what is next.

The certainty of an Autistic regarding their pictures is total. It seems when we try to communicate our thought to you it seems that you are not listening, don't care or simply you are ignoring the conversation. That's hardly a surprise as our thoughts are really complicated to you. If you said to me Grandma was nice or asked me if Grandma was nice? Our point of view starts with a picture of course, *say a thought picture of a kind Golden Retriever being petted,* (Remember we think in Pictures), I have several picture thoughts I translate 'nice' from. You have no idea were looking at a dog and relating how warm and bubbly its personality is while the entire conversation was talking of how nice grandma is. While our words also apply to grandma, as well as the dog, we are able to "communicate" the right things even if we had the wrong or odd point of view. Talk a little longer and it will almost a certainty that we'll loose you.

I remember in third grade telling dad how a light switch worked and the puzzled look on his face was priceless, I'm sure he was ready to scream but, he always kept his cool no matter how stupid the conversation. I was in reality talking of the electron flow through the switch; he had no idea I was "speaking atomic theory". Even if the thought had crossed his mind, his emotional thought would have told him no, "Rich is having a hard time in school what would he know of electrons." I was translating my picture thought directly from looking at the light switch on the kitchen wall, in the on position and just like the computer animation we spoke of earlier the electrons represented as dots moving along the wires showing how the current was moving throughout the circuit. I even figured out the resistance of the circuit in a motion picture, showing the electrons slowing down as they passed around the bulb filament. I didn't even get to mention that point to dad. Ironically, I realize the concept of resistance and seen it accurately in my picture thought, but figuring the numbers and using the formulas as you might do to figure out the resistance of the circuit is beyond me most times. As you can see one picture is worth a 1000 thoughts.

Another Point that needs to be made is normal thinkers are "Emotional" thinkers while an Autistic mind that never grew up on emotion is far more logical and needs a reason before falling for something, Autistics learn emotions after the fact. If people were more logical in their thought process Consumer Reports and The Washington Monthly would be the best selling magazines on the newsstand and people wouldn't buy solely based on the color of something. Keeping up Appearances would be seen as worthless. The concept of emotions dominating your thought is like pictures dominating ours. Look at the picture below, this is an old photograph of my Grandpa and his Model "T" Ford. I could easily see this picture as a thought picture for someone Autistic. Note thought pictures, are never in black and white but this example is. With a picture being worth a 1000 words this one is worth a million thoughts. Obviously not all million thoughts will be mentioned in our conversation but all will be based on it.

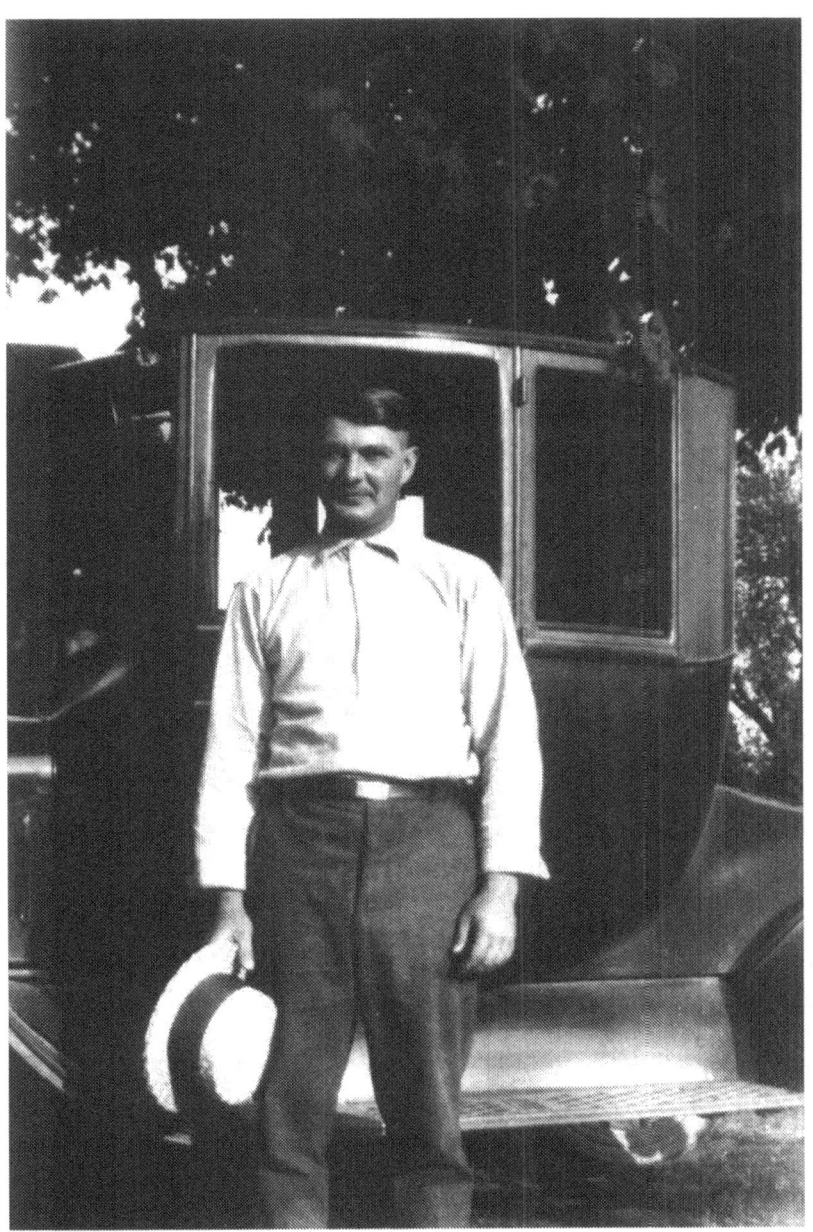

Rich's grandfather, dad's side taken in 1937?

Depending on what we are talking about, a certain point might be brought up. Hat's for example, obviously that is a summer one and made from straw. This hat in Grandpa's hand might lead to thought picture of more hats say a thought of a 50's era photo of men in hats, providing the conversation we were having was of hats. If the idea of hats were really prevalent next I'd see a thought picture of a store display I'd seen years ago displaying hats and the price tags. This photo would be as clear and crisp as the one you're working with now but in color. *From these pictures I could form the statement, "straw hats are inexpensive and typically worn on causal occasions."*

Other thoughts in the picture that spring to mind are 'the roof line' right above the windshield, from that I see a compete picture of Aunt Lottie's house. (Where this was taken) I'd have a quick millisecond picture of the house if the conversation was not specific to it, then it would be ignored. The little round mirror on the corner of the windshield reminds me for some reason of the stamping process that made it, including a picture of the stamping machine punching them out. Again I'd have a millisecond glimpse. While were on the subject of stamping the hood vents were stamped and my next picture shows the motor running and the air currents of the heat flowing around the engine compartment eventually escaping. That too would be a small glimpse. Watching the Weather Channel as the meterorologist explains the airflow patterns about the map is close to the picture thought I was having. In this case the motor might be seen as the United States in map form and the heat rising and escaping from it would be the weather patterns. Obviously figuring out all that frivolous information wasn't necessary for general conversation but it is indeed natural for me at least. Only in recent times have I been able to analyze the pictures/thoughts for what is needed.

Obviously, all along we were talking of how tall Grandpa was. Finally my mind would impose a ruler to him adjust it for the prospective of the photo and guess he was 5'6". This result obviously is pretty out standing providing I just "drew a complete house" seen a working stamping machine and a 'weather channel type of map' of swirling heat currents coming from the vents, all in a few milliseconds. I still was able to tell you how tall he was. Only recently have I taught my self to look for what the normal person sees in this picture, that being a kind caring man in the prime of his life. Inevitably, the normal conversation turns to how he looks like dad and me I suppose he does. *Please note the use of still and motion picture thoughts.* While I was doing all of this ultra processing I was too busy sweating the details trying to keep with the conversation to read or many times see your facial expressions or hear the subtle tone changes in your voice. In fact I probably didn't even see you 80% of the time I was looking at you. This indeed might play role in why we such a hard time identifying people. I have a horrible time recognizing people I should know, I'd have a hard time recognizing my best friend Doug if we met randomly in a crowd. Even normal people have trouble with that and you get more practice at it, since it seems you can take the time to read the face and hear the voice changes were not privileged to hear. Actually my final identifier at times is smell, quite a few people have a smell about them no, I don't mean body odor but unique "fingerprint."

A casual reference to a past holiday dinner could trigger an avalanche of pictures to an Autistic. The Autistic person might respond, again inappropriately, about an inedible cake served during that holiday. He might reminisce about the antics of a now dis-graced relative, not out of ill will, but because Autistic doesn't understand that these memories could be painful to others. The Autistic was simply processing pictures and reporting their content.

Today I make a conscious attempt to add one step to this translation process. You might think of it as a "filter program." If the pictures subject matter is inappropriate, I outline the subject in RED. I've trained myself not to translate into words any subject with a red shadow. This is where the name of my Web page came from, (The Red Shadows) my Red Shadow Translation Process. Referring to the Model "T" photo if Grandpa was a disgraced relative his out line would be in Red. The red shadow could just as handily be surrounding the window on the model "T," alerting me not to mention glass windows. (Maybe I broke one?)

So Far the talk has been a simple example of picture thought, one subject no distractions and no real pressure to figure something out. Plus I was probably in familiar surroundings where I was used to the tic of the clock and the noise of the well pump or furnace. If I were to look at the "T" photo while standing in line say at a fast food restaurant that was 'new' to me along with a noontime crowd I'd have a shut-down. Between the noise trying to figure out the menu my first two or three food pictures would be lost, all I'd see would be snow. Overload as it is called is like being suddenly blind and death for a few seconds. Eventually all returns too normal. In that situation I generally order a numbered special as there is less to communicate and I pay with a bigger bill than the meal cost. I trust the cashier to correctly deal with the change. Frankly, I do good to keep from having an overload in that situation and something as easy as counting money and having to process all that other noise and the newness of the environment all spell overload and shutdown. If possible I generally eat in the car where it is quiet and peaceful. Picture translation needs quiet and peaceful conditions to really be effective. After all were certainly doing 40 times more mental work than you are doing. It would seem the obvious gentle unconscious thought that guides you is lost in the Autistic process. Even though we think in pictures they seem to want to tell everything and anything with out regard to what the direct object might be. Like I said I had to teach my self to think along the lines you do, even if I have to do it in pictures. I can just imagine the trouble a young Autistic person has with this. I believe normal thinkers some times hear their thoughts? That 's strange.

Noise in excess is no more prevalent than Thanksgiving; the tradition in our family is eating at a buffet restaurant. Honestly that is about all I can handle. One year a lady with a high pitched laugh setting in a near-by booth drove me crazy. Dad was noticing the pain I was in when she laughed. I had to hold my ears. Typically I realize the general subjects we will talk about so they are "rehearsed" before dinner. I do real good in caring my food back to the table I really concentrate hard on just walking with out overload and the iniveatable dropping of something. I have had some small overloads while in that situation but nothing beyond handling.

I can generally handle crowds of 10–15 people providing I know most of them, and have a Q-tip in one ear (right one) to act as a hearing filter to cut down on the loud high pitched noises. I often find my self reading lips in those situations or referring to previous conversations I've had with that person, by doing that I have a good idea of what he said. Most people talk of the same things again and again. Even if they talk of something different it is in their same style.

Noise in general is as detailed as my pictures are, just I see too many pictures, and I hear way too much noise. Most people hear high notes but we hear especially high notes and about everything in between. While setting in the dining room of our 50's ranch house I can hear the clock in the kitchen the clock in the dining room, hum of the refrigerator and the freezer in the basement at times. If the TV is on I have a hard time "hearing the conversation" dad is trying to have with me: reading is impossible during that time. If I plug off my right ear things improve enough I can read. This is again noise-related overload. Every thing sounds the same to me the clock tic is every bit as loud as the refrigerator as is the well pump running in the basement.

I still wonder to this day about the "look" the school nurse gave me in 1ˢᵗ grade after she tested my hearing. I was in her office, undergoing a test with a mechanical device that produced tones. I wore earphones on and she was seated across from me with her control panel consisting of switches and dials. We did the low tones 1ˢᵗ and then climbed the scale and by signaling her with a hand gesture she moved up the scale. Finally I believe her dials were at their highest settings, I could even hear the buzz and hum coming from her machine. The noise was not coming from the earphone but was in fact blocked by them. As it made the highest pitched noise possible the look on her face was anything but normal. She sent me on way. I wondered several years later why I passed that hearing test and couldn't hear?

Even in the past year I did an experiment on noise and found out all kind of things. Many of you have heard the commercial for Mercedes-Benz motorcars where a deep female voice sings *"Falling in love again never thought I would…and the video is of the original Benz and progressively newer models.* For some reason I felt a need to hear and understand all the words to the jingle and thus recorded it on VCR 6–7 times in a row.

I listened to the string of commercials time and time again setting right next to the speaker, setting a distance away, and with the volume up and down and I still had a overload and missed the middle of the jingle. When I closed my eyes and listened to it things improved but it still wasn't perfect. Finally, as all "great discoveries" are made by accident I went to bed and accidently turned on the VCR: I'd left the remote lying on the bed and with my head buried in the pillow the jingle came through perfectly clear. BUT, If I looked at the picture I couldn't hear it. If I closed my eyes the brightness and darkness of the room filtered through my eye lids and I still couldn't hear it completely. But if I put the pillow over my face blocking out all light I heard the entire song perfectly clear every word. Of Course, I memorized it. Now that I know the words I hear it all every time I view it. And you wonder why a Sing-a-Long in an Autistic classroom doesn't do more than waste time?

Obviously, all of the inputs one has to process get jumbled up in the process in an Autistic mind. Its clear we can see, hear, smell and feel things (well even that is off a bit) individually but, doing two or three things at once really messes up the works. This suggests that the picture thought process takes up lots of brainpower. Processing everything including picture and sound from the T.V. didn't work as there proved to be too many inputs. Every time inputs were reduced the comprehension of the jingle improved. Eventually when all of the other inputs except sound were taken out of the equation, when my head was in the pillow, I finally heard the entire song. In my dream Autistic classroom blindfolds would be standard issue. The students could wear them as they see fit within reason. This might be a short cut to a lot of learning.

In Another noise experiment that I unknowingly done when I was younger; I had to start mowing grass. This in effect was noise conditioning: having the lawn mower motor running right beside me really made for an overall good experiment in noise and getting used to it. Today I realize I was running the mower motor slower than the average person would have ran it thus, it was quieter. Every squeak rattle and odd noise was instantly repaired or oiled: those odd noises were just too much to deal with. I can remember being terrified of the noise but putting up with it. It took me even longer to be able to handle the louder 2 cycle blowers and trimmers.

Today I wear super headphones standard ones that I have added extra foam to, they are really quiet and I can hardly hear the mower run when I wear them. I also put oversized mufflers on all the small motors we own. I also super insulate my automobiles; I had the Quietest Ford Festiva on earth, as I added sound deadening in every place imaginable. That Festiva had an entire 4x8 sheet of 4" foam in it placed mostly between the door and roof panels and the body. Think how small the Festiva is, in relation to all the foam that was in it. It was so quiet I often couldn't hear it run and had to roll the window down to listen for the motor at times. I really enjoyed the cooler months as I could drive with the windows all the way up. As an added benefit it was really a warm car in the winter. Driving that car on the road was a pleasure, as the noise was so much deadened that it was a non-factor while driving. It was even quieter than our house.

As you can see Noise is a major factor in picture translation. By controlling noise to the best extent possible other things improve accordingly. Basically doing a few things as possible at one time markedly improves talking and processing conversation. As Temple suggested in her book the computer is there, but, the processor and the modem are too small and I might add probably wired backwards. Somehow, I plan on getting a hearing filter, a devise similar to a hearing aid that block out many noises that cause me trouble. Those hearing 'aids' should really improve the quality of life. I have found good "hearing filters" are available in the form of hearing protectors sold in sporting goods stores (to be wore while at a firing range) that are rubber but feature a hole through the middle of them. They filter a lot of the objectionable noise out and still allowing for better hearing. I love to wear them in a crowd of people or while walking through a loud home improvement type store, finally I have a way to go into those hostle environments and still function.

Maybe since were using too much brainpower processing pictures the other inputs get lost in the process of communicating. Our normal picture thought is slow and time consuming and it is an accident if we somehow get the meaning of a conversation instantly. Even more unlikely, is the idea that we could talk about it, translate it, to speech in time to respond effectively in a conversation. Thinking in pictures is like thinking with a boat anchor tied to you. Noise, isn't a real part of the picture translation but it certainly has an ill affect on it. So far we have described in this reading the wonderful probably wonderfully smart Autistic person trapped in the world of his/her picture thoughts. I'll bet if the average Autistic person including the low functioning Autistic realized the thought process he/she need to create to interface with others and also identify some type of splinter skill or talent to which to learn by even the most challenged among us would markedly improve. This is precisely why we need an Autistic School devoted only to the Advancement of Autistic people.

This is the hardest and most complicated chapter of the book. I'm sure. It is however the key to Autism. I had to learn it bit by bit and I might suggest you do the same if this totally blew you out of the water. You probably have no other point of view to relate to so it will require an open mind to figure it out. The next chapter offers more explanation of picture thought. One final note on noise however, The first title of this book Perhaps You Have the Phone the Wrong Way Around—A Blind Backward Experiment in Autism refers to the trouble we have processing pictures and noise, When I came up with title I was thinking of a way the common person could experience to some degree how different our thoughts and figure out what is like not to hear correctly. Holding the phone backwards might be a close approximation of our poor hearing in bad noisy environments. Be sure to try this experiment with a friend. What you hear and what you miss will be representative of Autistic thought and hearing.

4

Day to Day

Autistic life as it turns out is quite an experience. I often wish I wasn't high-functioning as not so much would be expected of me, I was always brought up to put your best foot forward and do your best. Well, had everything been normal in my life that advice would have been really effective. The concept has really worked well in the long term but the Autistic perspective it has cost me several jobs. When I showed up for work on time dressed correctly and with a good attitude the simple job I started with soon became a springboard to something bigger. If I could consider my self-normal moving up would be an honor and indeed considered a promotion. However being Autistic and some what social I have a hard time saying no as it looks bad not wanting to move up in the eyes of the normal person but being Autistically drunk the typical promotion usually involves something faster paced and anything faster paced usually spelled trouble for me. Enchola, repeating a phrase or a word, is an ever present condition and somehow I have learned to hide that behavior: here of late my favorite word has been" Lucky" my dog that is no longer with us. Often times when I get the Urge to say Lucky I often have a picture-in-picture thought of him. The urge to say an enchola word is great and if I physically don't say the word at the moment my mind meant for it to be spoken I often have to say the word later when I'm alone. This is really a minor event however but occasionally I slip up and the enchola word gets out. Socially I have learned to brush it off with a comment of some type like, "Just Thinking."

One of my latest jobs was working for an Auto Auction, as was a stocker. Basically, I used a hand held computer and scanned serial no's of incoming cars. After scanning in the numbers and marking the options and recording the various account codes the car was entered in and you moved on to the next car. Despite the fact there was no training on the computer and the account numbers were never explained I caught onto the job easy enough. Standing all day however, was playing hell with my injured hip but pain pills were helping in that respect. After a week in that position I was approached by high up person in the firm and asked if I might want to go to another position doing the same job but instead of checking in the auto's on the lot I'd be doing it as customers drove them in. Suddenly the calm easy job had Autistic disaster spelled all over it. Now, I was working under a carport (echoes) and the cars were now running and each car had a driver that just had to in a hurry and insisted on screaming to others he/she knew. To make matters worse their were four aisles of running cars (horn toots and alarms as well) and 12–15 were under the car port area at one time. Besides the computer I now had a Walkie-talkie to deal with as well.

Suddenly, this job was an Autistic nightmare I was *drunk* trying to keep everything straight, the normal check in procedure, the new codes for this location and plus I now had to be the first impression of the company as I was dealing directly with the customer. All of this proved to be too much, I was having uncontrolled overloads (small ones) my 30% normal functioning mind was over worked and picture thoughts were more and more common. Soon I found my self tripping and stumbling while I was looking at a picture thought thus not seeing the real world around me. I even walked into a car. After several hours of this drunkenness I was sent for a drug test after I had moved a car from under the carport and got out of it leaving it running in gear! Thankfully someone caught it before it hit something! The truth be told I had just got a radio call and was thinking of the answer and just found my way out of the car. Normally I'd never leave a car running let alone in gear.

Well it so happened I had taken one of my Darvon (1/2 tablet) the day before as my hip was hurting and it indeed showed up in the drug test, and when I could not produce an Rx for it I was fired. I was put into this position since I made a favorable impression with the manger there as I presented myself well and they thought I would make a good impression with the customer. No I didn't have enough forethought to tell them no (Autistics think in slow motion) and by the time I realized I said yes I was in too deep.

My best long term job more than 4 years was washing mini buses. That job was kind of invented by me I had started work driving those buses and found that it was too much and since my employer never had a bus washer that had worked out I took over the job. I worked totally on my own set my own hours and came and went as I seen fit. It was mostly evenings and weekends and I washed 30 or more buses per week, as well as ran an occasional route and delivered buses to drivers that had become stranded when theirs quit. I also did a little rocket science there by fixing a mechanical problem no else could fix, one that stranded the whole fleet at times. I had invented a test and a cure to fix a broken fan belt problem that plagued the newer buses of the fleet. Sometimes the belts would break once a week and soon they were being replaced once a week: that was the mechanics official cure. Autistically I knew the problem was not as serious as it was being made out to be and the wild fixes that were not working, never even came close to identifying the problem, in fact it was made worse with every new fix. Everyone thought the pulleys were out of alignment but in reality there was too much stress on the flat ribbed one piece fan belt and it was no longer running flat. It was in fact running in a rainbow pattern wearing the edges of the belt eventually causing fraying and eventually the belt broke or jumped off it's pulleys stranding the bus.

My test simply painted the belt with normal white paint and after it dried one started the motor and as the paint wore off the center of the belt returned to the normal black color first. That meant the belt was riding up in the middle. In fact one belt I tested was left on the bus for another few days and when it broke the edges were still white, meaning the belt never ran flat as intended. Austically I realized this was the trouble but I had to prove it to the mechanic which was twice as hard as it normally would have been. One I had to break down the barrier of the mechanics ego gracefully and to I was out of the closet. Mechanics don't take kindly to being told no matter how gracefully what the problem might be: worse yet by someone Gay. He did think highly enough of my work however, to plagiarize it. I'm told he pocketed a large bonus. Of course, I didn't help my employment either when I sent pictures to the main headquarters of "on the floor brake pedals" and bald tires.

Eventually, my job was abolished when they hired an outside firm to wash the buses. It was just as well as I had just suffered the injuries form the falling axle and I was to the point where standing was a chore let alone washing 30 buses. I often received two christmas bonuses and I was liked by all the employees and clients but management was not quite as delighted. In fact if I hadn't been their best bus washer ever I'd been fired years before. If I were in the same position today, with the added experience of knowing about Autism and learning from it I could have handled the events better and might have been able to get credit for my work. But, as I said before the best ideas in the world are void when coming from an Autistic person that hasn't learned the way the real world operates.

My other long term job, (2 plus years) working in a department store as a sales clerk, It went really well and I received several positive customer comment cards from it but after I was outed with the events surrounding my co-worker Mike's death I was accused of "stealing the store" and fired. I was told years later by the security guard in question who was then working for another firm that it indeed had been a set up. It is called cleansing in the retail trade. The deeply religious roots of the store and it management for sure played a part in the decision to get rid of me, no one (openly) Gay could work for them.

In current times I find employment much easier to handle providing I choose my job correctly and it if is stress free and I work alone I can do wonderful these days, proving it isn't full time offering insurance. I recently had such a" good" experience and all was going well till the 90 day trail period was up. Soon I was being warned by staff members and clients alike to "be careful". Soon like at the retail store I was accused of stealing and fired. I later learned through the grapevine that my Autism was revealed in the insurance report. When I priced insurance on my own I was blown away when the premiums were going to be $5000 per year. No employer paying someone $7.00/hour is going to spend that much on insurance for one person. Ironically, everyone according to our states department of insurance must be eligible for insurance. They don't mention anything about the price, however.

Personally, I don't have trouble at all being social and developing long-term friends and as I said before that aspect of things is a lot easier dealing with "family" other Gay people. I generally find people ok for the most part but I have had several instances where Autism or the label of has been worse than the condition. Generally the comment is "retard" etc. I was actually once asked Why, I was driving (had 1-800 Autism sticker on my car) and why I wasn't in a group home, like Rain Man? Others don't like to hear of my insurance lack of care stories. Many very ignorant people think everyone is covered under welfare and that welfare is really a working safety net. I've been horrified the number of people that respond to my Autistic web page and get all worked up over the fact I'm Gay. I have had two page e-mails from parents of Autistic people telling me where to get off. I have actually been able to get some of these people to talk of Autism occasionally but as Dear Abby told me every time they communicate with me a little bit more of their ignorance is enlightened. Even if I don't agree with someone, I was taught to respect his or her thoughts.

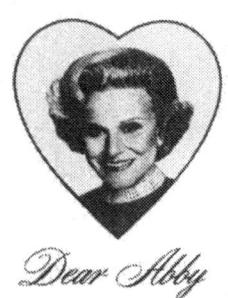

Dear Abby

Dear Rick,

Even those respondents whose
verbal violence to your website has
prompted your letter, have had a small
degree of their ignorance enlightened.

Whether or not they disagree 100%
they have been exposed to the thoughts
contained therein -- which may be what
they are referring to when commenting
that they will not allow their children
to browse your site.

The best advise I can give you on
how to reply, is to do what I do. Take
each communication and respond to it as
if it is the first time you have seen
that point of view expressed, while at
the same time allowing your past experience
to inform your reply. As you know by
reading my column, the human condition
is repetitious, and each and every one
of us views our own issues as unique.

Thank you for providing me with
new and valuable information on Autism
and its impact on Gay lifestyle.

All good wishes,

Abby

Today I'm not at all shocked to tell my readers I trust very few people, after a close acquaintance of ours who by the way was the first to preach to me and tell me I was going to hell for being Gay, re introduced himself to me in a sexual way years later after learning of the Autism. I suspect he thought he could get by with something in light of all of those 'advantages'. I had more than enough self-respect to tell this person to get lost. I suspect he sets in his reserved Church Pew on Sunday and is forgiven. A lot of homophobia often stems from people that are Gay themselves and hiding it or possibly someone totally ignorant of the whole concept of being Gay. As I mentioned before the ignorant often resort to just plain intimidation to make their points.

Otherwise, Living Autistically requires a lot Planning and pre planning something weather it be an appointment or a trip to the store always takes some serious thought on my thought. If it is an appointment I have to rehearse in my mind every possible scenario so that I'm prepared for the possible questions. If I have just recently viewed the possible picture thoughts the day before the moment before, I can often think with out the pictures. But if I'm passed a ringer as talking about something I was wasn't expecting to hear I'm instantly at a dis advantage. Of course sometimes my pre throughout scenarios allow me to pre-suppose the wrong things and get the wrong meaning of the conversation. If Someone has to be a "Funny Man" and joke and kid about everything that usually confuses me especially if I happen to see a few of their gestures or facial expressions, and they don't relate well to the thoughts at hand.

Even family affairs are a tight experience. I'm really proud of our group family photo and in it I'm wearing 100% goodwill clothes and even the suit jacket which started out brown was converted to black when I spray painted it. Well there was no need for cologne, during the photo shoot but more importantly it looks respectable and the money saved was used for better things than a one-time use event. I'm so used to living on a tight budget that even the simplest of things like helping a friend do something sometimes wipes out my entire budget if I end up buying some simple mechanics supplies or have to buy string for the trimmer. Life used to be easier when Grandma was living I was always her "pal" and she made sure I had the funds I need when I did something big. Even when I was working money was tight but grandma had been through the Depression and loaned me some of her frugal living skills. I even have taken them a few steps farther over the years. I know my family always tries to include me in their events but I feel so guilty sponging along many times not having enough money to leave a good tip if we go out to eat.

Especially in the past few months now that our lifetime family home has been sold: things have really become serious. I have been on my own with out many of the advantages I once had living at home. I no longer have my A-B-C ordered garage to work from and the common oil change is now an event. More importantly I lost my best communication partner my dad. I no longer have anyone that lived with me through all of those 911 events and seen just how difficult life can be for a square peg. I lost the only person who understood my picture thought enough to talk to me in picture thought, he sometimes say, "I bet that made for some real interesting picture thought." The biggest thing I have to deal with these days is the injured hip; it prevents me from doing some of the jobs I'd be good at. Of course, treatment for that is something only the privileged with health insurance can accommodate. I'm sure I'll be able to find something somehow that I can be good at that pays well enough to earn a living. I even was reduced to 'bread and water' for a few weeks when I had a budget crisis when I had to fork out some money for unexpected auto repairs. Even pawnshops are a common event these days. Well, I'm not complaining I have many wonderful moments and have many more experiences than many of my Autistic counterparts. I'm just glad I can be happy with the simple things.

Moving out has put me into various living arrangements in the past few months and Luella and my A-B-C ordered shop as well as my furniture is now crammed in to 10x30 storage facility. Despite being perfectly organized it is just too tight to even attempt to do auto repairs in it and I'd never want Luella to set out. Besides it has no electric and the no one is allowed in after 10 at night. I still somehow manage to take advantage of my splinter skill to work on my daily driver but it is a chore.

Dad had given me when we sold the homestead his old Toyota Previa and even Toyota 's wear out and recently the I had to replace the Alternator and the official Toyota part was beyond my budget as was any part since I had just paid the car insurance so I found my self in the junkyard making a "New Alternator". Since the Previa has many one of a kind parts due to its odd but dependable design many of the interchangeable internal parts don't directly switch from one car to another. The alternator was no exception so I was forced to build a new one sitting the junkyard parking lot that unitized the Previa only parts and the "new" more generic parts that would interchange. Junkyards are typically in poor neighborhoods and this one was no exception. I was forced to build the alternator right on the junkyard lot as dusk was setting in and I'd been driving all day without the Alternator thus I was running out of battery power and driving after dark would have stranded me when the battery finally went dead. Anyway, while setting on the dirt lot working on my alternator I was now alone as all the employees had gone home. Being Autistically unaware of my surroundings I never even heard (but I heard the click, was listening for the click of the brush holder to seat) the robber come up from behind the van but I did feel the gun on my neck. Of course, I didn't panic my Autistic mind was too busy to really figure out what that gun was capable of and just how unstable the person holding it might have been. I simply lied down on the ground and counted as the robber fled with my wallet. After a reasonable amount of time I was kind of relieved to see my wallet was still on the lot and everything was in it but the cash. I quickly finished the repair and burst into tears when I started it and the Alternator light on the dashboard was out.

That wild event didn't even seem to register with my family. I wonder to them if was just another unbearable Rich event. My odd medical stories, my mechanical adventures, being fired for being Autistic with a $5000 insurance policy attached to you and being kicked out of the hospital and doctors offices for lack of money and being too odd, make a hold-up look like a walk in the park. After all my family has seen all of the strange stuff I have done and they're probably relieved that no matter what the event is if it doesn't involve them they are happy.

Besides these event the simple process of moving out has been a horrible event to itself. Losing the family home an all it entailed was not unplanned but still the shock of it all produced 4–5 nervous breakdowns on my part. By that I mean I just became so overwhelmed that I lost control of everything that happened, I couldn't think or function without just crying and my nerves were shot. My normal Autistic conditions were highlighted in a more obvious way and I really realized with that experience just how much different my normal state of being is compared to someone else.

The move out forced a lot of things, Luella Mae my old tailfinned boat that was a real sight when towed behind my old Pontiac was donated to the Larson Boat Museum. That donation really struck some of my family members the wrong way but they failed to see my point in getting the relic to a good home where it would be preserved and they also failed to realize the typical buyer would probably turn it into a fishing junk. When I had acquired it was just such an item and it took me two summers to restore it to some presentable condition. It also would take resources beyond my budget and skills to bring Luella Mae up to showroom condition. Maybe some day I'll be able to see her again in the Museum.

Life does have its good moments despite all of this, I enjoy the Lambda Car Club events and going to the P-flag meetings in my old home town even the simple 40 mile trip to Lancaster takes some planning some months if the budget is tight. I have on occasion had to drive all back roads to the event so that I could run around the speed of 30 MPH where gas mileage is the best and I could improve it even more by coasting down hills with the motor off. By doing this I have enough gas to both do the P-flag event and get to work the rest of the week. I really don't think Grandma intended me to be quite that frugal.

In some respects that Group Home that I have despised so much through out the book sounds interesting at the moment but I'll make it on my own and would rather do with out like I typically do than live in one. Besides I probably function way too high to even be considered for one.

I'm indeed thankful that Dad never gave up on me and I realize he has earned his retirement and the traveling it will entail and this is as good as time as any to break the connection. I'm not all that shocked that some friends and family members are kind of distant and I understand their apprehension about taking dad's place. Simply reading this book my readers get a good enough idea that I wouldn't be quite the perfect house mate as most everyone would be a polar opposite of me.

5

Schooling and Education,
It was not in the Text book

Kindergarten started September 6, 1966 for me. I was the youngest kid in the class of approximately 20 and it was a ½ day session. The experience turned out to be the first of many bad education experiences and if you will a forward looking mirror predicating what was to come. I had no preschool. It was here I learned I couldn't skip use scissors with any control and in general my progress was concerning all involved. My education, the strange adventure began here. Hopefully, my experiences can go a long way in resolving a lot of Autistic education questions. Remember, my education was void of official Individual Education Plans (IEP'S) my plan was simply that I didn't learn or grasp something and mom and dad seen to it I was tutored. The IEP's of todays special education system kind of sound good but, coupled with the entirely wrong learning environment for someone Autistic the best IEP is deficient in that aspect alone. The ideal school for someone Autistic would teach picture thought, in a well disciplined quiet school, with out a sing-along. As you're about to read I unknowingly did it the hard way.

In kindergarten I received the first of a pile of notes sent home for mom to see concerning my progress, if I'd kept them the entire stack might be several inches high. They were especially common through 3rd grade. Something must have really been askew, as it seemed these notes were tied directly to the new events that happened in class. Occasionally, I received notes for doing something correctly, usually that sparked hope for mom and dad but the good events always happened later for me than the other kids.

The "forward looking mirror" effect was really illustrated early on in the first few weeks of kindergarten. The teacher had hung on the wall a card board cutout of Mother Hubbard's Shoe and the names of those able to tie their shoes was listed in chronological order. Initially I had been listed in the forth or fifth place but, when I had to demonstrate the ability to tie my shoes in class I did it backwards, maybe this was due to overload as I remember everything getting QUIET and I thought "just finish-up" so the people around me would leave. Yet, I was tying my shoes at home? I was removed from the list. It wasn't until the end of the school year that I finally made the list, last. That "Quietness" might have been my first recognized overload.

About the same point in time during a summer visit to Weldon's Ice Cream Shop in near by Millersport Ohio, (Buckeye Lake) I had another overload perhaps my first one out in public. Weldon's Shop sets right on the water front and features a long "Grand Hotel "type porch and the building its self makes for a natural reflection of the noise traveling off the water. Well to the normal person that is no big deal but in my case leaving the shop and walking down the long porch holding two Ice Cream Cones was something beyond me. I remember being blank-walking in a blackness void and somehow getting to the end of the porch and nice lady talking loudly finally getting my attention and telling me we don't hold Ice Cream Cones sideways as the Ice Cream fell out of the cones and on to the porch. Indeed we didn't hold them sideways but when I walked out the door I was intrigued and baffled with the noise of a passing motor boat and the echo it was making while passing the shop going full speed. The noise of the boat was just too much to deal with and somehow I kept walking. The dropped Ice cream was just chalked up to being a kid, but I was puzzled for weeks what had really happened and even recall practicing holding stuff the rest of the summer in an effort to figure out that event. At the time I was ignorant of Autism and never realized we kind of use only one sense at a time and the sense of hearing was definitely being overworked. Today I wonder if the senses are closer to normal but, processing what the senses are doing by the slower picture based Autistic mind is just too slow a process for anything close to a normal pace.

While doing research for this book I ran many types of educational checklists offered today as a guide to see if one should be tested for learning disabilities. I suspect that if I were given a checklist in 1966 if such a thing existed I'd showed a clear need for an L/D education then. But, again that would have only lowered the standards I would have had to achieve. Over the years I really by accident, improved most everything on the lists to an acceptable level. But initially, at least I'd tested poor in most all categories. If I noted it in my research notes I lost track of the author(s) but I seen several versions of this in various items I read.

Generally speaking some list offer coordination as a first checkpoint. Instantly that would have been the first clue, I couldn't skip in kindergarten, through out school it was proven I couldn't run fast, do jumping jacks or Swim really effectively. Except for the Jumping Jacks and skipping which are still beyond me, I have found ways to get around the other misfortune. I was really athletic in my younger days and found I could do slower paced sports well. I took up bicycling and have ridden some 8500 miles in my lifetime. Golf was also a past time as well.

Reading ability is mentioned as another point to ponder, It was never great the Dick Jane and Spot Readers I grew up with were somewhat easy I thought, maybe it was due to the picture content. However, Mom and Dad were worried that I wasn't getting the point of the story and I remember them working with me almost nightly. I think if anyone had an idea I was thinking in pictures or trying to they would have seen the sudden a bigger reading problem coming when the picture type books were phased out of the curriculum. In fact some of my first tutoring sessions were for 3/4-grade reading. Suddenly having to read with out pictures highlighted just how much I was relying on pictures in first and second grades. Of course over time I have learned to read both Autistically and in a more normal way. Simple, really simple things can be read with out picture thought, but more complicated things are read Autistically and converted to normal thought and speech.

Complex instructions are also a checkpoint and still troublesome to this day, mostly due to the picture conversion (Autism) process, having to read or hear the instruction convert it to pictures for thought and then act on them is a time consuming process. Sadly, quick picture thought does not lend its self to keeping the details of complex instruction straight; thus sometimes-obvious details are missed or ignored. Even today the obvious information that the normal thinker takes for granted like the cursor on a computer screen moves left to right and the enter button makes it work sometimes needs to be explained to someone Autistic. Add to this a little bit of dyslexia that I have also overcome and the simplest of directions become a chore.

Lists go on from here to include Attention spans, For the most part it has been endless I never give up on a problem until it is solved. Autistic distractions such as noise and processing many things at once might sideline a thought but generally won't void it. However, the glazed look, often exhibited by Autistics are probably not inattention just the physical appearance of us looking at our pictures. If one hasn't developed his/her pictures yet they might be looking at a "blank picture" but never the less their thinking.

Memory for letters and words can be a real problem B's, p's, j's, d's, f's, l's 2and 5's z's and all get confused for one another when I'm in a hurry. Memory for words is better has always been a problem, mostly from an Autistic point of view, and the fact there are pictures associated with words and the pictures need to be "looked up" and associated with the word. Multiple words meaning the same thing are a real chore. For the most part during my early years I had a single picture single word vocabulary which was really slow and needed to be precise. Over time I started using random pictures to decide what a word means and then simply checked the content of the message to see if I got the right idea. This is a much faster process and only occasionally when I guessed wrong does it affect things. If that happens I need to redo the picture thought process.

Some of the research showed some L/D lists questioned one's ability to tell direction quickly. I still have trouble with instant left and right if I'm involved in a something fact paced, but for the most part it is not a problem. Growing up in the country, was a great teacher for the sense of direction, I daily watched the sunrises (east) and sun sets (west) and even got to the point where telling time from the sun's position was accurate. That daily lesion really developed my directional ability. Today I apply that sense of direction to my picture thought and hardly ever get lost while driving. In fact via my Picture Thought (computer animation) I have the ability to impose a moving dot on a map when I'm driving to a new location. It is just like the new high-end cars with the navigation systems.

Handwriting is even on the checklist of nearly list I referenced, as well it has never been great but slow deliberate writing is fine but normal writing like my notes I wrote for the writing of this book are almost unreadable and filled with dyslexia type of mistakes.

I love the organizational parts of the questionnaires. I now have my entire workshop is in alphabetical order. This was a learned trait and one that was much needed. Necessity, in the form of those volumes of picture thoughts need some type of order: thus my life is now in A-B-C order. I needed to do that in grade school, but there again no one knew I was dealing with volumes of pictures. As for the answer to this question I was not good at organization.

Since of time is also considered; These days, as always, I'm early for everything, I really have to think about time questions or any involving the order of events: if I don't I'll get the story incorrectly. As for Social interaction and Timing in them that is not quite so good. This is indeed a sore point but Thankfully I had some of the best friends growing up in school that alerted to me to my social blunders and were kind enough to give me pointers. This Gay "Charm School" has really helped. Sadly picture thought and all of its translation doesn't often keep up with normal conversation thus the inaccurate poorly delivered statement isn't always that intentional.

Are you popular? Do you want to be why not? This is listed in many books as failure of one to become social and join clubs and participate in sports. If you get nothing else from this book, get this Autistics are not "You" and shouldn't be expected to be you. We spend a lot of our energy just keeping up translating pictures and just plain figuring out our world, frankly were too tired to worry about a popularity contest. Sports for many of us especially those with coordination problems is out of the question, gym class is bad enough. Maybe some types of after school functions might work for some but as a rule I'd bet the Autistic would like nothing more than simple peace and quiet after school. We might engage in some odd play were so famous for. Once a few things are figured out Autistically, I predict there will be a spurt of social growth. Suddenly one will start worrying about some social things. Please quit worrying about eye contact, it will come naturally someday. If we are not making eye contact, I suspect something autistic is going on.

Finally the best is for last, the ability to think for yourself; believe it or not we have that ability, but since our lives operate in slow motion thanks to the slow Autism conversion process, we often can't think fast enough to do little more than get in to trouble. We often end up with de-fault answers, a yes or no or a suggested answer just to keep the conversation flowing. I have found in real life this inability to think fast has got me volunteered more than once to do something I'd normally never considered.

Well I've been the lucky one I blindly figured out a way and a means to make the best of Autism, thankfully along the way I had the best of parents and the best of tutors to make it happen. As I finally developed socially I was ordained in the Gay Community as part of my Outing Process and Gays and Lesbians and the Transgendered I met who had been well bashed themselves often were most tolerant of my social blunders. If I were straight I'd needed to have been surrounded by their tolerance and love. Typically, a person that has never had to deal with xenophobia (fear of persons who are merely foreign) in any form reacts to it in a negative way and most importantly refuses to deal the problem, weather is the oerineration of someone or the strange behavior related to a mental condition. Had I been forced into the straight community at large I'd been called an idiot and shoved into the misfit category (I still get called that in the right circumstances) and never given the pointers or the chances of redemption.

Just like kindergarten, being up front and backward at the same time I was like this through out school and college I often realized what I was doing long before I could demonstrate the fact on a test or in person. When I was at an after school tutoring session one-on-one with someone all seemed to work much easier. Almost every tutor told me you knew this, why did you come here? The hindsight answer is I did know it, but I had to figure out a way to get from my Autistic mind to a normal one. Kindergarten, turned out to be a lot of stuff, the experience of being away from home was, as bad as, school itself. Figuring out one couldn't skip or use scissors was a puzzle for even me. Other kids were doing it? I should have been able to do so to. Typically kindergarten kids were more tolerant of one of their classmates not being able to cope and I was even encouraged by many of them to keep trying. That helpful attitude never completely faded away throughout my schooling but in later years I was quite the oddball. It is also helpful to note the small rural country school and the general attitude of the era (Mayberry RFD) also played a big part in one person helping another. In Fact, when moving to the real school building for 1st grade, each class was given a lecture on school etiquette and we were instructed to treat the Special Education students that we now shared the building with equality and with respect.

First grade was quite a challenging in a number of ways. From an Autistic perspective my teacher Mrs. Nutter had a beehive hair cut that made my head "spin" just watching it, I was always looking for a swarm of bees to invade it at any time. The first cloudy rainy day really proved to be an alarming experience as well, suddenly the room was getting brighter and darker. Of course, I was seeing the cycle change in the florescent lights, something only Autistics can see I'm told. I still remember the puzzled look on Mrs. Nutter's face when I raised my hand and asked her why the room was getting brighter and darker. I think she thought I was referring to lighting striking. Now days the lights are phased and the cycle changes are not there to notice. Once in awhile I run across a light that isn't phased but it a rare event. Autism was unknowingly playing a part in the 1st grade experience as well.

I do believe my first still picture took place in first grade in reading class, a group of us were reading a picture book of some type probably Dick Jane and Spot and we were doing an assignment where we were to find objects "hidden" in a tree. I was having trouble finding the objects the others had already found, BUT I did see a picture of something, spot or a dot where my present day picture-in-picture thoughts appear. It might have been related to the lesion that I might have seen before in my Dick Jane and Spot book. I had no idea what this odd picture was about or where it might have come from. I remember the class and those setting beside me NOT being there when I seen this small glimpse of a picture. In retrospect, It sounds like an infant Autistic thought. The rest of first grade was the typical torture of knowing something and being lost, notes sent home from school. Finally the use of left-handed scissors. (I'm left-handed) really helped my cutting ability. The famous hearing test I spoke of in a previous chapter where I flattered the nurse by hearing it 'all' also took place in first grade as well. I was never held back in any grade, but I was considered for special education more than once I'm told. Thankfully, mom and dad worked with me at home and got me through it.

Second grade continued much as first grade had and in third Mom and Dad sent me to a place in Columbus Ohio, called Reading Research Foundation, it is similar to The Sylvan Learning centers of today. I went they're for an unbelievable amount of time, to me, and in reality it was only two or three months. I was tested on all kinds of things, all kinds of ways and finally we quit going. I never did hear of what the official findings were but as your about to hear again I'm glad this was 1969 and Autism hadn't been heard of yet in most circles or I'd been diagnosed then. IF I had been I would have been put in special education and I feel my progress would have been severely limited. After all, the aim of special education isn't exactly the best thing that can happen to someone Autistic.

The Reading Research part of this Autism experiment in passing turned out to be a futile attempt relative to the times of finding out what the trouble might have been in someone's education. Kids having trouble in school were sent to this place for a strange mixture of army type discipline combined with exercises (testing coordination?) and classroom stuff including reading tests. The results of the performance were supposed to identify the trouble one might be afflicted with. But in 1969 Autism wasn't a buzzword as it is today. In doing research for this book I attempted to trace down anyone that owned or worked for the firm but it ceased operation in 1974(?), that is when it disappeared from the city directory. I was in hopes of finding official records of the place they might have been helpful in determining today if I'd tested Autistic then. I was also intrigued reviewing the official letterhead of the business that several of its key persons had the titles of Lutenant and Sargent? Maybe some of the students attending the foundation were more of behavior problems in school than anything else. One note the best things happened here: when I was blindfolded and a soft voice did the speaking. Today that 'lack of using all the senses' really relates well to Autism. To bad we didn't realize it in 1969.

I also learned while writing this a friend of mine also was sent to the Reading Research Foundation three years after I was and he to had similar stories of the army type discipline and the general torture of the place. His problem turned out to be dyslexia and they never came up with idea either. It was his mom that finally detected it, even though he went to a Catholic School.

Socially school was progressing; most progress was forced interaction. Recess for me was spent most of the time setting alone of in one corner of the playground, no I wasn't lonely in the least, I was using this time to catch-up on what I missed out on so far in that school day. I remember being a comfortable distance away from the rest of the screaming kids. Occasionally, I did the swing sets but that was the most I ever did. Of course I was in no particular hurry to demonstrate my odd physical abilities, by this time I figured out I couldn't run with out falling over.

As mentioned in the Picture section fourth grade brought about the first for real still picture, If only I'd known what to do with it and all of the others to follow? If I were a parent or teacher of and Autistic I'd tell the student that one his thoughts are different from normal and if he sees things, tell him those are his thoughts! Coax him to use those thoughts, by describing them to you and most importantly what they mean to him. Odds are they will make little sense to you, but tell him so in a kind way you don't understand. He will eventually find a way to communicate his thoughts, it might take awhile be patient. I could also expect to hear from the student "Pictures?" I don't have them, I really didn't have them either until fourth grade. Prior to that I had some small momentary glimpses of something I sometimes thought of as blackouts. When I discovered these were really connected to my thinking, I started 'finding them' and looking at them.

Oddly, I ignored them once I figured them out, maybe since they really didn't relate to the thoughts at hand as I seen it. As I mentioned before I continued to ignore them until eighth grade. But, meanwhile I was using the book A Charlie

Brown Christmas as I described earlier to figure out how things were working via pictures. I never admitted to anyone that I was even looking at the book, let alone using it on a daily basis.

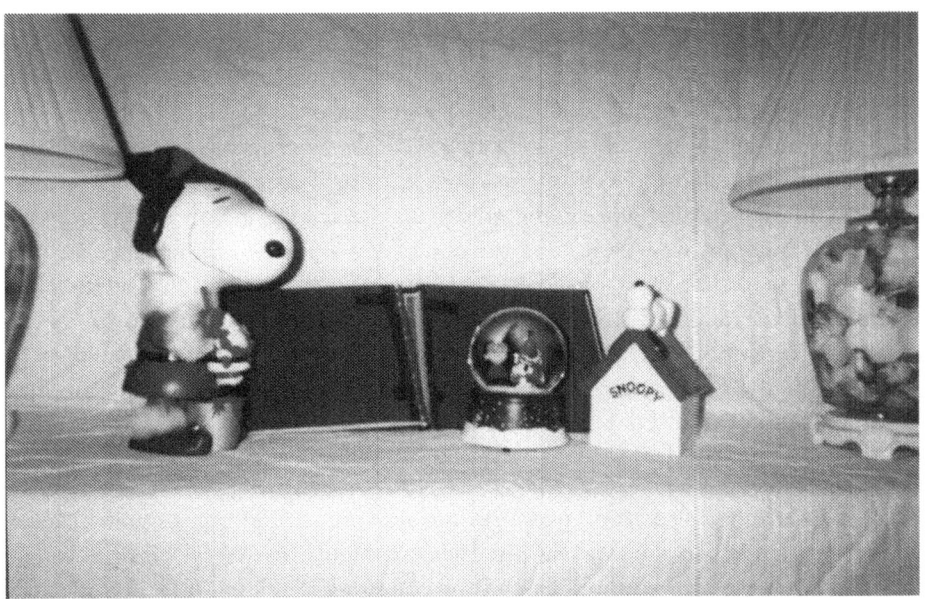

Pictured is the well-used Peanuts book.

It was unknown to me taking the place of the pictures I was trying to ignore. Looking at that book is how I learned to translate pictures. During this time from a normal point of view, tutors mom and dad and even the teachers discovered that if they tried to teach me through my obsession which was cars I did lots better at grasping the idea they were trying to push. I learned how to divide numbers by figuring miles per gallon, a little bit about ratios by figuring the gear ratios in a car and even the color chart was learned via cars. "If a blue car hit a green car the resulting new color would be yellow." Actually, my pictures were geared toward my obsession and since I had already figured out a good deal of the Autistic "interface" dealing with cars it was easier to deal with new ideas in the same vain as the old ones. Learning division on the chalkboard in class was terrible as I hadn't developed enough 'math interface' to figure out how to communicate it. Plus math in general for me is really hard anyway, with out the common interface to communicate the ideas I'd really been lost. I bet other Autistic's could learn a lot, realize a lot, if they were taught via their splinter skills.

By the time I made it to Sixth grade school was still pretty much a pleasant experience as the same small group of kids that were with me in Kindergarten were still my class mates and friends, somehow I was still liked by them any many tried to no avail to include me in their lives, but by this time I was realizing just how hard it was for me to handle the developing social aspects of life. The girls in the class were staring to dress up, and the guys were developing their own personalty and traits and suddenly the simple reading, writing and arithmetic was accented by a popularity contest among the students. Guys were in "ah" and "keeping score" of which girl was developing the quickest. I was too busy figuring out the three "R's" to realize they were coming of age. When we lined up for the class photo that year all of the Guy's were trying their best to get near one gal in our class that developed early and they all had the hot's for. I for one was just as intrigued by the guys as they were with the girls. That experience was somewhat puzzling, but thankfully I was to distracted by Autism to worry with the sexual oerineration.

Seventh grade and the start of gym class and moving to a different style of classes where we changed classrooms was just about too much for me. All that noise, in the hallway while changing classes and the banging of lockers all made for a real experience. I found myself carrying more books than needed so that I could spend as little time as possible in the hallways during class changes. Even then the noise was too much. Gym classes that started that year were alone responsible for a number of firsts. One was my First major overload where I seen snow screen and seemed instantly 'not there' one second and back again the next. This is where I couldn't do jumping jacks. Since then I have spoke with several Autistics on the Internet and have discovered many have similar trouble. I only have that trouble when fast rapid movement is necessary, so fast paced sports are out of the question, but I can do the slower things like bike riding (well I used to) and golf. Today I can actually play baseball and I couldn't in school. Just like driving, If I keep in normal thought mode (no Picture thought) I can follow the ball and actually hit it.

The overload in gym class was almost daily and the echoes were really the major cause of it. The gym was and echo chamber and every squeak of a shoe on the wooden floor was heard at three times as the sound bounced back again and again. Plus the noise I naturally heard beyond what the normal person heard was creating a bigger problem as well. Looking back I realized unknowingly for some months due to my keen hearing a loose board on the gym floor as it squeaked when it was stepped on. I had heard that squeak for months prior to the floorboard finally giving away. The girl in the ladies gym class that was hurt would have been most grateful if I told someone as her leg was cut up when it gave away and her leg was trapped. The basketball was always bouncing too often and a few shouts and screams were all that was needed to spark an overload. The gym teacher was always screaming at me to tell me what he had just told the rest of the class. I had been having overloaded and never heard the instructions given. Even until the end of gym classes in 10th grade I never could do a jumping jack. The Gym teacher pulled me aside and tried and tried to get me up to doing them but finally gave up. I would hope in this modern age the clues of no skipping, running and now being unable to jumping jacks might be taken as signs that one is not normal. By now with the advent of the classmates being my friends was fading, soon the whole school knew of my jumping jack problem and starting with junior high the population doubled when students from another part of the district joined us. Suddenly all kinds of new friendships were being formed and enjoyed. Only a few of the old crew still spoke with me, and that was more of a obligated kindness, since our parents knew one another as much as real friendship.

In eighth grade when I experienced my first motion picture and I was really amazed at it my self. Where did it come from? Why was it a perfect image of the inside of a car motor and why was the motor operating in slow motion. Finally I figured with information like that those pictures really did mean something. This was the first time I really questioned weather my thoughts were really similar to the average persons. Socially, I was really losing touch, other kids were worried about whom they were being seen with and how they were being perceived. I on the other hand could have cared less. Fortunately, for me mom any my sister 'forced' me to wear fashionable clothes thankfully or I'd really been a nerd. As the kindergarten mirror predicted, In junior high and high school I was on the honor roll a few times and at the same time I had to take algebra 1 again my sophomore year as I didn't grasp enough of it in my freshman year to move on to algebra 2. Even in the second year of Algebra 1 I never made a better grade than a 'B'. Most of the marks were 'C's.

In my sophomore year I experienced my first easy class ever; environmental biology. This class went well I feel because it lent itself to pictures easily, as the teacher talked of something I had experience with. I just had picture after picture of related picture thoughts. There were no math concepts in the class, and growing up in the country I had already experienced many of the concepts of what the class was discussing. In fact my pictures went back to earlier times working in our garden, and walking through the cornfields where I learned explored and inquired on my own, long before that class. Plus, having a crush on the teacher didn't hurt either. Strangely, that was very first time I really ever was attracted to a person and the Gay part didn't bother me a bit but I was puzzled finally figuring out in 10th grade what some of strange social behavior displayed by my classmates was about. That turned out to be the end of my home school education experience I spent 1–10th grades in the calm, quiet town of Carroll where everyone knew everyone and the cop was "rented" every weekend. Somehow, It was decided that I'd attend Vocational School the next year in the near-by town of Lancaster and it turned out to be another challenge.

The Next Step Vocational School

During my junior and senior years I attended a vocational school in the near-by but yet distant town of Lancaster. This was a 16 years olds dream come true, I had to drive to school everyday as no bus service was offered. The trip was 15 mile one way. I can honestly say I learned more of life driving to school that I did in school. I learned through experience how to drive without brakes and how to call others help when the car died. Autistically bashful, it took an act of courage for me just get the nerve up to call home when something happened. Understandably, being different and unknowingly learning on my own in my own way I had grown quite independent. The first time the car quit running and I had to call home for help was a real experience. Many times after that when calling for a tow truck on my own I often had to dial the call 2–3 times before I'd let it go through. Autistically confused I was trying to get my thoughts together enough to tell someone of the trouble and describe to them where the car had stopped this time.

Anyway I was enrolled in drafting class and I quickly learned that the pictures a draftsman drew were not really art! These were precision math based drawings: that took the fun out of it. But, even though I never did real well in the program, I really enjoyed it. I often had dreams of the popular "Xerox" copier commercials of the time (78) where the Monks were using the copier to do great things, quickly. I was always puzzled why my perfect pictures I had in my picture thoughts could never be duplicated by my hands on the drawing paper. I even wanted to pound my head on my drafting table a couple of times in hopes it might act like a rubber stamp and simply appear on the paper. If only that would have worked, I'd been at the top of the class. Of Course the picture thought was stimulated with this type of class and again if I'd known what was really going on and had a better interface with the world at large I'd made better marks.

Otherwise the new environment and the tripling of the student population really worked to my advantage, I was no longer known as "flash" and my social blunders were not as noticeable in a class of 900 or so. Plus no one had any idea of my past and the reputation that went along with it. I actually did find time to be social on occasion and it was kind of nice to be liked in some respects. Plus the entire aspect of the school was much more liberal. There were social groups never heard of at my old school and even a group (unofficial) of gay students. Everybody would have been in the closet at my old school. Looking back I found one of the reasons I was popular was the fact I drove ODD cars to school Luella our 62 Pontiac was an admired car by the guys and when it quit running the substitute transportation was a 61 Chrysler with HUGE tail fins and George Jetson styling. If I'd had the rest of what it took to be a social climber I'd made it pretty far along.

I had a reputation according to my drafting teacher of being a good boy, but little did he know I was leaving school at lunch sometimes to drive downtown to the car wash: I always had to have a clean car, after all it was Luella I was driving, and the Autistic as you might be aware gets more attached to objects rather than people. Luella was my best friend. I later learned the local school deputy sheriff had known I was going down there but he too thought I was good kid and besides he liked my old car and the fact I was caring for it, thus he let me slip by time and again. Probably, in some ways I was really doing myself some good, totally getting away from school for awhile. I was lucky I was never in an accident or the car ever quit running or I had some explaining to do. I had no real idea just how much trouble I'd been in.

As it was I did get one detention in high school as my senior drafting teacher had placed me in between the two loudest people in the class in an self admitted effort to get me to participate in class, At least I'd have to say shut-up to both of them thus I participate in class in some form. It really worked well as the two on either side of me were having one of their conversations despite the fact I was seated between them and I finally had enough and yelled shut-up. The ultra religious teacher took offense to it: I had a detention and I was the talk of the vocational school for a day or two. Between my picture thoughts and the added trouble of being in the middle of a conversation I didn't want to be in, it was just too much.

Otherwise, School went ok grades were great to horrible and mom was really horrified to learn via a call form the school in the last weeks of my senior year that I might not pass the Civics class and thus not graduate. She hadn't had any alarming calls from the school in years and I indeed was ready for a break and just got lazy during the last days of school. At the time it was hard to explain to her but I did manage to get enough points to pass on my last test.

The Diploma actually came from my Home school in Carroll and as such I had to go through their Graduation Ceremony. It was for sure interesting returning to the school I had so "lovingly" learned to hate. I was instantly greeted by the old nickname Flash.

If I hadn't realized how different I was in high School, College certainly pointed it out. In high school where your life was still regulated to a large degree the structure I think an Autistic mind needs was in place. College however, was missing that structure and in reality no one really cared if you showed up or not to class as long as the tuition was paid. This gap of having to provide your own moral support and take responsibility was not hard for me, but it was like flying alone in relation to high school. I think many Autistics would have trouble making the switch.

Through the Aid of a local Scholarship I was (for I'm most thankful for) offered by the Wagnall's Memorial I was able to attend college and Technical school. Student's living in a particular township graduating with a "c" average or better qualified for the scholarship. I had one quarter of college and had chose the major of computer science only to find the math to be far beyond me. The only real enjoyment of the college was the history class I had to take. I should have known for sure, from that point on I was different—I was the only one in class to remain awake during the whole class and further I enjoyed the class. I was indeed watching the "History Channel". My pictures simply flowed with whatever the professor was talking about. I hardly looked at the book and the test was easy in that class as I simply glided through my pictures and answered the questions. Others in the class thought I was on a "happy drug" seeing as how I enjoyed the class and done well in it.

After my quarter was over, and I realized deep inside I'd never be able to handle the calculus, I went against the wishes of my family and enrolled in auto mechanics school. This was an associate degree program and indeed the most rewarding experience of my education. I easily aced my auto classes and for sure looking back I was getting more out of them than the rest of the students were. I think all the drafting experience really paid off as I seen lot more to a drawing or a picture of a part than I should have. Picture thoughts and the related engineering drawings provided by my picture thoughts made for another positive but not quite correct learning experience. While my classmates were just learning the basics and thus just becoming parts replacers I was having an engineering experience. I became one of the elite few people in the nation that really understood the car. Even Henry Ford was ignorant of the motors he created The leader himself, was lucky that some of his first motors ran. Thanks to the Engineering based professors in the course everyone in the class had that type of experience shoved down their throats, clearly many of the mechanic type people in the class thought it was too technical for them. I for one enjoyed it. I think I'm one of 10 or so people in the nation that calls a motor a vacuum pump and fixes the simple stuff first and lets the high tech take care of itself.

I was somewhat dismayed that I tested so low in math on my entry exams that I was placed in remedial math class. This stuff was even easier than the Algebra had been but still it was a chore. In my other classes I did ok in some of them; chemistry was my downfall. I took it four times and had many different tutors and still I couldn't pass it. I understood the basics likes dissolve likes etc. but when the math and the Periodic chart had to come together I was forever lost. It is the only class I lack to complete my degree. I tried and tried with tutors of all types and even though I didn't mean to I even confused them. In all my years of tutoring, I never confused a tutor until now. This was a reflection of just how far college chemistry was beyond Autistic thought. The last chemistry I had had was in junior high science class and it wasn't nearly as in depth as this.

Besides the chemistry class, I made one of my first major errors in my life I had signed up one quarter for advanced English something by Autistic accident. I had tried to schedule standing in line at the registers office and in error (lots of noise and commotion in the room) crossed numbers and ended up in the wrong class. I was two weeks into the class before I was pulled aside and told I was in the wrong class. Oddly I was doing ok in the class and would have passed it. After leaving the class standing in the hallway collecting my thoughts I got to hear the professor make a few snide remarks and the laughter of the former classmates brought back the bad memories of gym class, thankfully the thick skin remained. I really felt super confused and lost for the first time in my life I even skipped school the next three days and spent them in a daze wondering just what had happened. After that event I felt so lost and out of touch and I really didn't even know who to tell about it. I had always lived life on the fringe but this is the first time I really fell flat on my face.

As far as Auto Mechanics went I was in bliss working with and doing my favorite thing; working on cars. But the bliss ended there. If I'd had realized the fact I was Autistic I'd seen the poor choice I'd made in a career choice as my shop experiences pointed out I was in the wrong place to work safely. The shop at school was a modern state of the art, car repair shop. It was quiet clean and fume free and it was even quieter than the gym at school had been, all giving me the false impression all shops were on this caliber, I had little overload trouble in this shop. But I did experience a few close calls here that again should have served as fair warning. In Brakes class I had dropped a shop light and broken the bulb and I was too busy thinking and looking at pictures of what I was doing next to realize that I had started un screwing the broken bulb with the POWER ON. The sudden gasp and then quiet of the class finally alerted me that I was in danger and not a moment too soon! I had known better than to play with electric and would have never dreamed of doing such a thing. Like wise through out school I was often being yelled at to move, get out of the way etc. Unknown to me the small overloads I was having prevented me from really be 100% aware of what was going around me. This not the place to be Autistically drunk—being a little death dumb-founded and blind for a few seconds here and there.

I went ahead and went to work in a garage without the degree and soon found I was really out of my element in many respects. I could fix the cars others only dreamed of fixing, and at the same time I never got along in the shop as I was always having overload and the real shops were far from quiet and perfect. I was always being yelled at and being pulled from danger. And here I though my only trouble related to the fact I was a stereotypical klutz at times.

Personally, as a result of not graduating college I was having a terrible crisis as I had to deal with telling my family that I couldn't graduate college because the classes were to hard, that was like admitting that you had killed the Pope or something. I never realized until recently that they wouldn't had been surprised to hear the truth, but admitting to the fact, I wasn't able to pass-was to me admitting failure. I still have a dream of passing the class and earning the degree: Since

I now know of my Autism and have put my thoughts in ABC order I feel I could pass it now. There again the Chemistry is really a process for this picture based mind and I might not be able to even now pass it. I have grasped the ideas of chemistry, likes dissolve likes etc. but the numbers and the formulas that make it happen is beyond me.

College also included one trimester at DeVry (elcetronics training) and it to was very easy and hard at the same time. I also ran into math trouble there as well. After realizing the math involved I gave up on the idea in just one trimester. Once bitten twice shy.

College in general proved to be my outer limits in terms of undiagnosed Autism and its effect on my life, in retrospect I'm glad I made it that far along but, still it was short of what was needed. Oddly, in work and in real life no one realized I didn't pass college and many thought my mechanical skills were the result of the college but I suspect college only served as a vehicle to expand my already present abilities. I feel I'd be doing the same thing in the same way even with out college. Granted it might have taken me longer to get to where I am now but still I'd made it.

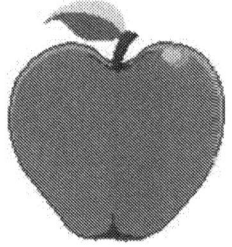

6

The Autism School of the Future

You wouldn't dream of sending your kids to a school or pre school that didn't have a numberline or the alphabet displayed over the chalkboard. Every teacher would need to be totally qualified, nothing less would be tolerated! But yet in the Autism school we would feature a Picture chart to go along with the ABC's and the number line and most importantly teachers that understand picture thought. Kindergarten teachers would teach our baby pictures like they teach normal kids how to say letters and count. Grade school teachers could tell us of how to use and develop our still pictures and begin a process of telling us how to turn our autistic thoughts off an on. The science of Autism is simply Greek and currently misunderstood by even the best experts. That is simply an invitation for massive ignorance, and the wild and sad state of Autism education is currently based and treated like typical MR/DD. If it were Autistics would have no success at all, as this type of education doesn't trip enough switches to make us anything but irritated. Once Autism figured out I predict most folks would be mainstreamed by 6th grade and quite a number of us would be able to drive as well. It had been done time and again in an era before Rain Man and with a little insight from the best of today's education there is little reason why we could not turn Autism into a 6-year "Latin" preschool. Even Behavior issues would be easier to deal with when Autistic thought is controlled correctly and our senses are blended into the education process.

Autism 101 Development of picture thoughts from basic to the advanced

The Following Pictures are the very core of Autistic thought, they start with our baby thoughts and wind their way up to our most sophisticated thought that trumps even the best of normal thought. Perhaps it was the sophisticated thought that Alan Turing used to develop the computer with? Maybe some of the great thinkers of our times were picture thinkers to, some one had to come up with the idea the world was round : Picture thought would have been most suited to that problem.

The photo below *is as normal as we are going to get!* This is the same thing you would see if you were standing right beside me. This picture will be the goal of all Autism, a picture like this indicates normal thought. Normal thought is much better at hearing and seeing smelling and does not mess up as easy. IF WE learn to control our Picture thought, normal thought like this is 'useful'. It takes some work and practice to get normal thought to work for us. Please note, the lack of eye contact everyone seems to worry about probably takes place during Picture thoughts like these.

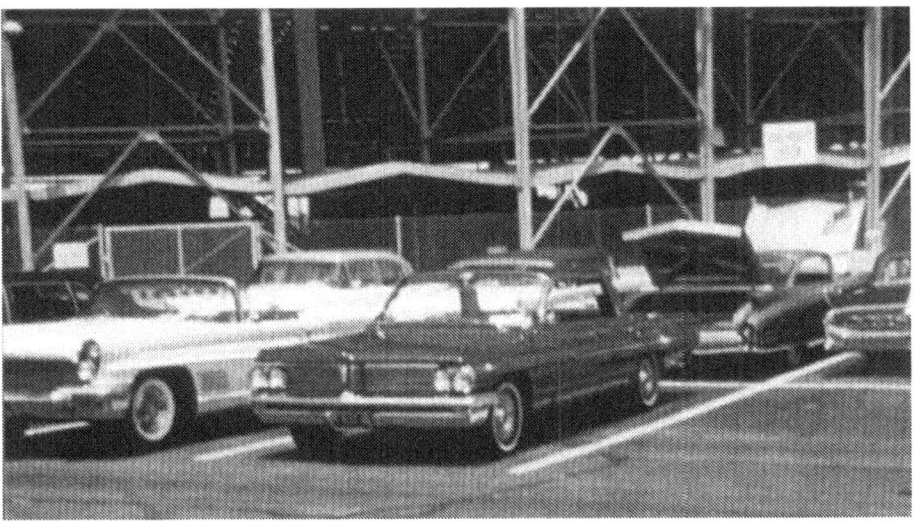

*Figure 1 We are seeing the same thing! In real life and in the picture
thoughts to be explained*

All Picture Thoughts are in color. The Publisher of this work could not do color photos.

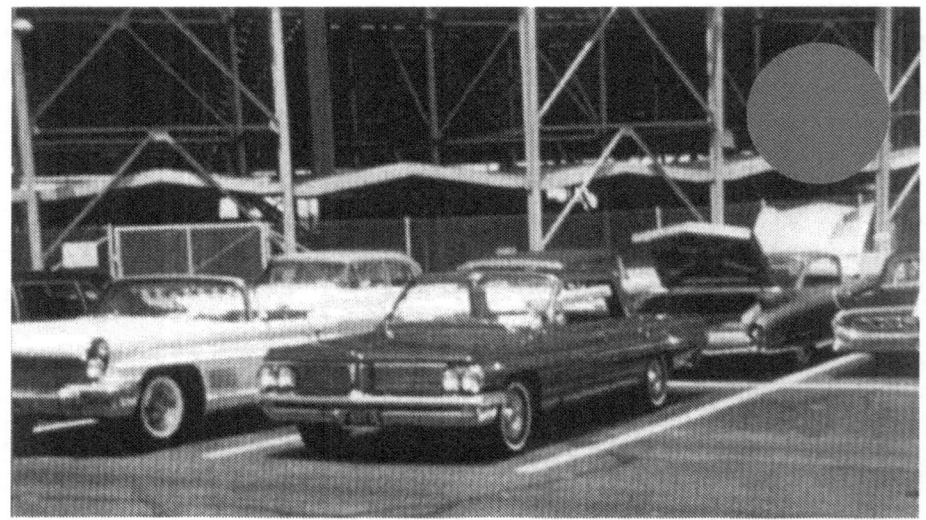

Figure 2 Now, it is a baby Autistic picture thought.

The Blue dot represents an actual Autistic picture thought This Spot is created by the brain and is probably displayed with help from the optic nerve. In reality it is not blue but more like a 'black hole" This is indeed one of the first steps in Autistic development. The Autistic classroom needs a picture like this to tell our kids 'this is expected' Autistic teachers need to know this to. This spot occurs naturally, and I often wondered Why I seen All of those Spots?

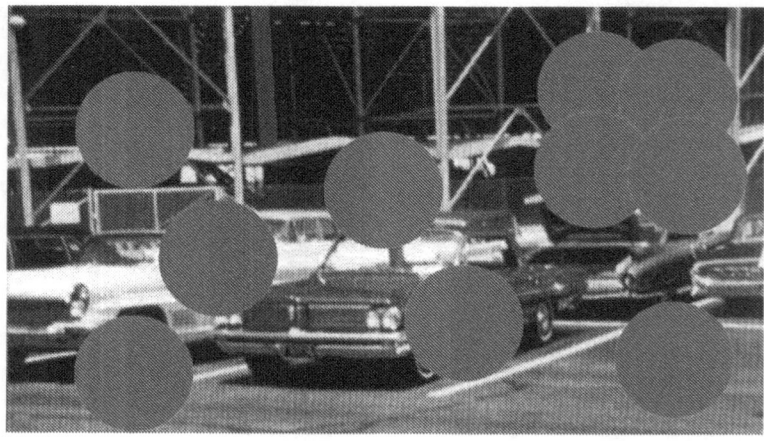

Figure 3 An early baby thought from kindergarten, All of those spots!

The single dot in figure 2 never settled down from this instantly. At times when (hindsight) when I was having my first picture thoughts they were all over the visual field, just like this all at once. Perhaps my brain and optic nerve were having a fight on where to put it or how many spots to display? Eventually, I don't know how, the dots simply settled in the upper right hand corner of my visual field. I remember asking the question quite often, Where did all of those Spots come from? Why, didn't anyone else talk about them? Finally about 1st or 2nd grade the spots became one dot, the one in the upper right hand corner that I still use to this day.

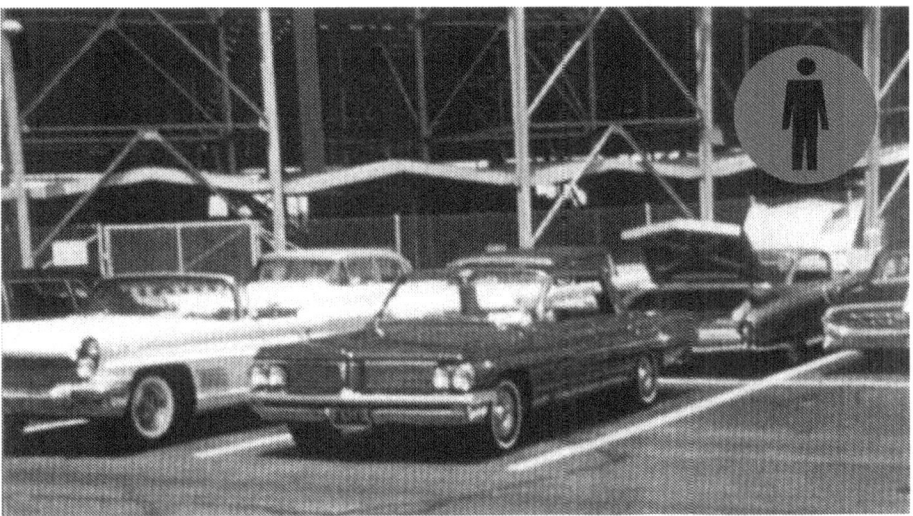

Figure 4, The dots started 'communicating' things, pictures appeared in them.

Sometime around 1st grade, the dots—later to become thought pictures-started displaying pictures. Most of the time the pictures were unrecognizable but some were of simple things like stick figures (above). Eventually the pictures became something I could figure out. One my first was of my little green Huffy bike that was one of my favorite toys. Eventually I thought they might have been of people I knew and place like home, but no one was talking of thoughts like these? I tried to desperately ignore those Dots and for sure, I quit mentioning them to others, I was already a borderline "something" and talk like that was an invitation to the funny farm. If I had known those were my natural thoughts I'd embraced them instead of ignoring them. As it was I was often yelled at for not paying attention or daydreaming, most of the time it was due to the fact I was looking at that little dot trying to figure out its picture. It was finally in 4th grade I had no choice but to pay to attention to it! That dot became my first full size Picture thought. ***The blue dot simply 'blew up' canceled normal vision and took over my visual field!*** My Optic nerve was shorted out, this 'dot' picture replaced normal vision! See Figure 5 below.

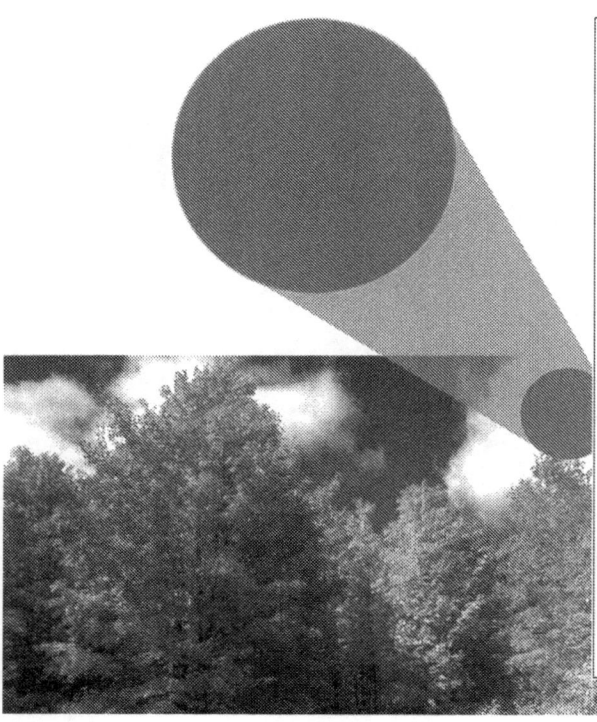

Figure 5, The Blue Thought Dot took over my visual field! It simply jumped from its corner spot turned OFF the optic signal from the outside world and replaced that with this thought.

The classroom lecture was of trees changing colors in the fall and in the night before reading assignment there was a picture of a tree changing colors. This was the first time I had seen this picture. As the teacher started talking of the assignment that picture re-appeared in my mind again canceling out the optic vision! I was Stunned, where did everyone go? I no longer seen the back of the heads of others or the teacher or chalkboard.

Quickly the Picture Thought disappeared and soon normal vision returned. The Red Car in Figure one would be gone, replaced with this mind imposed picture, and soon the Red car would return when normal vision resumed.

Oh Boy, What an event! WOW I'm on this thought trip and I didn't even leave my seat in the classroom, thank goodness I was not walking or something. After the shock of the event itself, my brain tingled for a few minutes afterwards, possibly it was the connections being made, or the realization of my natural thought process. I knew better than to scream out in excitement or joy that would have only added to my strange aura.

This was indeed was my first real picture thought, If the world was geared and understood the Autistic mind at work this event would have happened years sooner possibly in Kindergarten. Now I started paying attention to those pictures and the little dot pictures. At this point the dot pictures started to mean a little more. I still didn't have solid thought pictures and it was another few years before I had another one that canceled out the optic reception like this one did. Still, no one else had thoughts like this, my little dots seemed to just mine.

Finally 4 years later in 8th grade I had my next thought canceling picture thought, just like the one here the optic reception was canceled out completely. This time the picture was like a cartoon, in many respects IT MOVED IT was a motion picture!

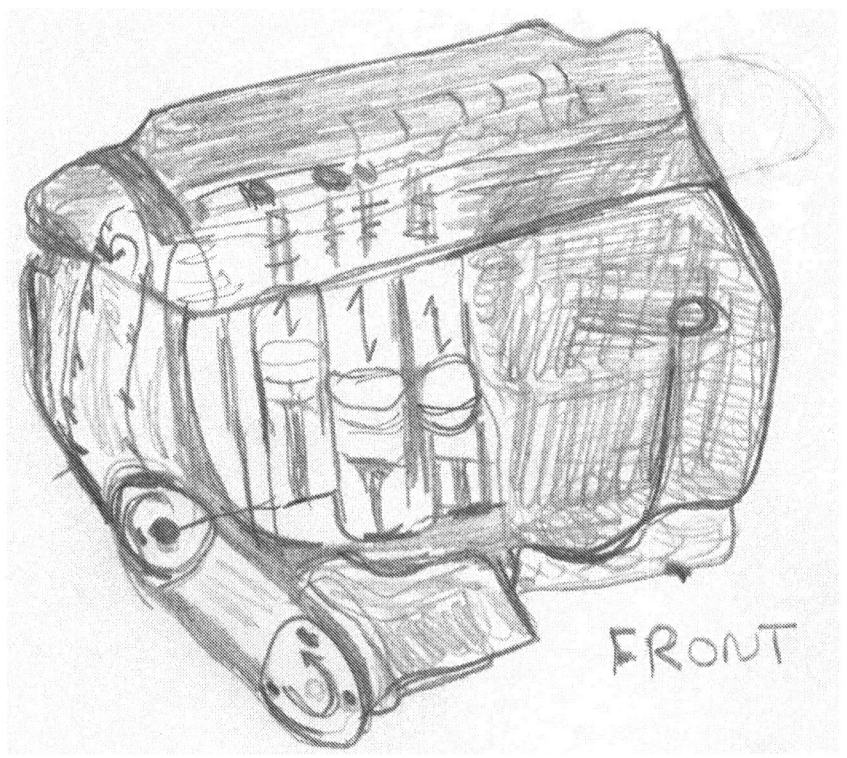

Figure 6; imagine this picture in Motion! Running if you will, it was doing just that in this new motion picture thought! Note I'm autistic NOT artistic it took me hours to get this engine drawing this good. The one I was viewing from and comparing to in my Autistic Picture was 1000% crisp, clear and accurate, just if I were looking at it in a Polaroid Picture.

Life Simply gets better, now there is yet another picture that cancels out optic reception and this one moves! This new picture was as puzzling as the one in 4th grade was. As before The teachers lecture prompted the event, he had been talking of combustion and mentioned the light part of it was unnecessary, as you couldn't see inside the motor anyway. Well, I could? Thankfully I kept my joy to my self and stayed out of the funny farm, yet again. This time as before my brain was a buzz with tingles feelings etc. and prior to that I had felt good but remember being notably tired when leaving the science class that day, It felt like I just ran 10 miles. From then on I decided those pictures did mean something and I had better start using them. If I could have told someone about the picture, I could have easily filled a 25-page report ranging from the oil to the strength of the crankshaft, the overall design of the motor and even the number of links in the timing chain. I knew all of that stuff from the picture but had no way of telling anyone all of that information. This is where converting Autistic thought to normal thought takes place. As it was in school I was barely making C's with the help of a tutor almost nightly. Just think if I could have UN trapped all that autistic knowledge and written that report? I would have got an A for the entire year.

Now the fun really begins, it turned out these picture thoughts were just first steps, possibly first steps a few years too late in the total picture. I had been trying my best to ignore them after all. The next picture represents the next picture thought process Picture-in-Picture thought.

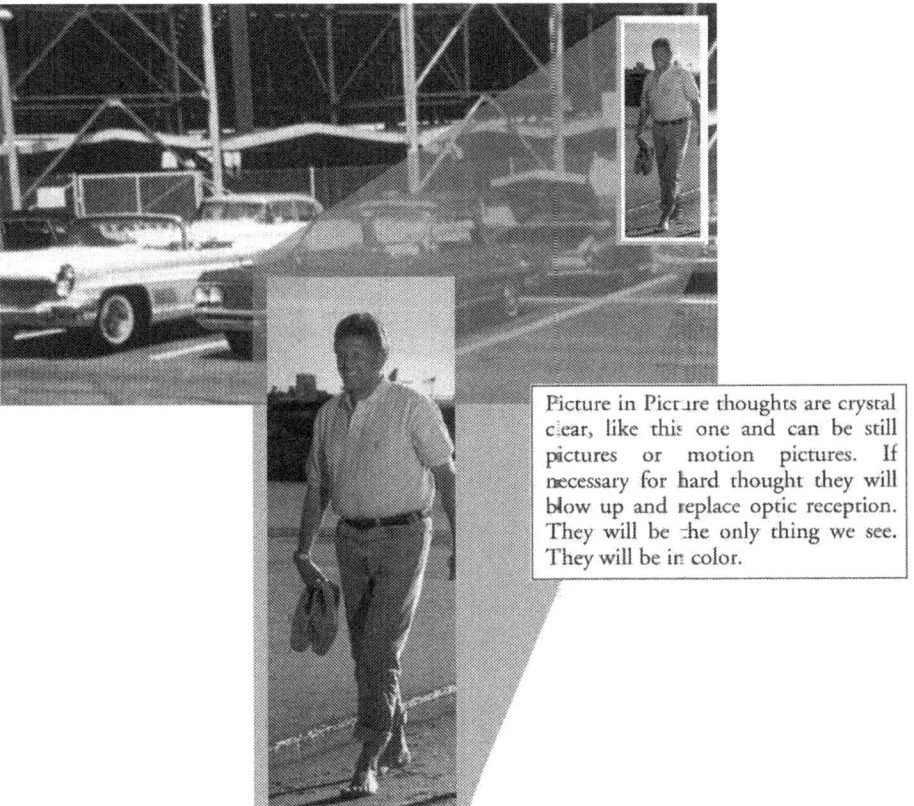

Picture in Picture thoughts are crystal clear, like this one and can be still pictures or motion pictures. If necessary for hard thought they will blow up and replace optic reception. They will be the only thing we see. They will be in color.

Figure 7 This is Picture in Picture thought.

After the Big Still and Motion Picture that canceled the optic reception these small picture in picture thoughts finally started making sense and the pictures were no longer blue dots but real intelligent pictures. The little picture sometimes showed the number 45 for example telling me what page something was on. Sometimes a motion picture would show me walking to the bus telling me (showing me) if I locked the house on the way out. Often times the picture in picture thought is a combination of Motion Picture and Still thoughts. Anytime something needs to really thought about the Picture in Picture thought just cancels Optic reception and all I deal with is the Thought Pictures. During this time all the senses seem to be turned off and go into the ROIT (recover) mode meaning it takes a siren to wake up us from our Thought Picture. The picture thought probably takes up 95% of our brain power thus the last 5% of our power is used by the senses to keep us alive. It would take a loud bang, the quiet wisp of something to alert us to impending danger and return us to normal thought. The world gets quiet no matter where we are. Sometimes if were trying to process the picture thought and keep up in the real world everything goes blank or we see snow screen indicating major overload. What I wouldn't give for a Pentium 4 processor in my brain. I have learned over the years to control the Thoughts of all types, this is dangerous thought to have if your walking or driving obviously.

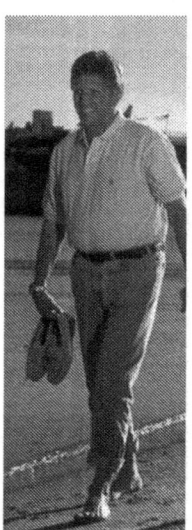

Figure 8 what is in a Picture thought?   Everything!

This Picture thought could be a still picture, or a motion picture, ex, the guy could be pushing a snow thrower up the driveway. Or like this one a guy walking down the beech, We can glean from this the temperature, the weather, who this person is, is he a relation? , What is a polo shirt? How tall is he? How much does he weigh? Especially when dealing with people sound s can be a part of a still or motion picture but for the most part they are sound free. Smell (fingerprint) often plays a role in Identifying people to.

Note ALL PICTURE THOUGHT is in COLOR!

To make the sentence," Stan was walking down the beach holding his shoes." We indeed might see this picture in our thoughts.

To do the sentence ,"Stan was walking down the beach at Four PM. " we might see the this picture and one of a clock or our watch or even get an idea by where the sun might be: hold a little piece from each picture and translate it to a new sentence.

Now life gets complicated, there are 1000 words an a million thoughts to go through before any of this picture can be come speech to be spoken. There is Conversion process that takes a bit of the thought picture and converts it to speech. If there were25–30–50–150 pictures in a thought a little bit of each thought (picture) would be stored and soon a sentence to be spoken would be formed. This is the "Latin" Autism conversion process. That takes inside information of being there and doing that to know about. UN-trained Autistic thought naturally wants to tell everything the picture has to offer but typical conversation and the normal person could give a hoot less if the chimney in left side of the picture was made of 14,000 and some bricks and was shortened 3 foot when it was recapped. They don't care if the driveway is Blacktop, concrete or gravel or someone is walking on a beach.

The Normal person is looking for the idea it is cold/warm there is only a little bit of snow or a lot of beach, and the hot chocolate is probably ready. It would take the Autistic picture based mind some time to come to that simple conclusion with out some training.

So now we have the development of Autism it started out as little spots that were actually primitive thought. No one had a clue that we were not crazy if we mentioned them. We sat in school and ignored them and soon the idea of Full size Picture thought woke us up or tried to. Then we have Motion Picture thoughts that also tried to convince us we have a different process in thinking. Finally about 8th grade we get the idea there really is something to those pictures. Meanwhile we learn to think using both normal thought and Picture thought, and develop way to control both. Soon Picture thought can keep up with conversation and lots of simple normal thought becomes routine. We learn to look at a picture thought and make words from it.

In real life I bet the Autistic is using 95% of his or her brainpower processing those pictures, think of the trouble a slow computer has on a webpage with lots of pictures on it. That might be why everything else doesn't work unless it has to. The LESS sound we hear, the less we see, and even the less pain we feel would tend to conserve brainpower for its normal functioning. The 5% we have left has to keep us alive, works by being extra sensitive, If were doing Picture thought and walking at he same time I'm certain it could keep us from walking off a cliff but it will not guarantee that we will not look like a FOOL.

It took a lot of hard work in regular class to push and develop our regular thoughts and flip enough switches to trigger our natural Autistic ones. I doubt any of us would have made it, as far as, we have if we never forced in normal classes. I wonder if the modern Autistic was ever forced to learn anything? For sure Picture thought was never taught.

For the moment we could start teaching Autism in some form or another like I just described to our current students. We would have to tell them they think in pictures and if they see Spots work on figuring them out. I'm not sure the picture time line I presented is typical of Autism development or just a version of my warped luck figuring out Autism. But none the less we need to start thinking and talking pictures. Our kids will have to be our best guide to tell us if they are grasping anything of Autism or if they are learning to think on their own. I have faith in the fact of the past people like me and before me all somehow learned

Autism and made the best of it. NONE of us knew what we were doing but we did get a Ph.D. in Autism. If we did it on our own, I see no reason the best of modern education couldn't break a few molds and start over when it comes to Autism. If were really diligent we might actually get this whole Autism thing figured out by 6th Grade. After all Autism is mostly a second language with a few twists none of which are not insurmountable.

As for teaching, the "new "Autism, once teacher and parents get the idea there is a different process going on here they might want to drop the typical education standards. Once Autism is figured out and allowed to blossom a bit we can go back and fill in the blanks. If some one has a splinter skill or an obsession, RUN with it. That Splinter skill is a hall way into the Autistic mind and short cut to all kinds of things. The Splinter skill amounts to a ready made interface that might take years to develop if it was never pursued. You might have a young person fond of Trains (thanks to an Autismtalk.net user for ideas on this) so do everything possible you know to do that relates to a train. Have your student learn of steam and how it is made and how it works. Have him/her learn to count by counting the cars on a train, teach them of time and schedules by teaching them train schedules. If there is an interest in circles have them learn of train wheels and learn math and geometry by figuring the radius and other things via the train. Have them learn of electric and diesel motor in the engines and compressed air that is used to stop a train. Take an obsession even further by having them research what trains carry and where some of the countries are that the goods come from. Have them find the countries or states on a map. Eventually all of this One-track knowledge will simply spill over in to common life. Really stretch it to the limits by showing them an old movie where people traveled by train and point out how they behaved and dressed. Remember I finally learned division by figuring miles per gallon on a car, to do it normally was torture as I had no interface developed for divisor, dividend, quotient etc. and numbers were never a strong point to begin with. But I could tolerate them long enough to figure out something about a car.

Otherwise, we need a place all our own like a deaf or blind school. It needs to be QUIET and debical meters need to be installed to give everyone a chance to experience what the Autistic is hearing. We need labs that help us discover what normal is when it comes to our bodies and pain tolerance. We need to figure out what a normal person feels as lite or what qualifies as heavy. I remember breaking almost every bolt I touched as a beginner auto mechanic; MY Tight was another person over tight. I soon learned by using a torque wrench what 20-ft lb. felt like to me at least. It felt like I barely tightened a thing. We might have a supervised Weight lifting class to further tell us what should hurt so we learn when to quit. Yet another lab might videotape our encounters so that we might get an idea what picture thought was cutting off our senses and view of the body language of others. We might be able to begin controlling our picture thoughts better if we knew how it was adversely effecting our performance. People watching us could finally be aware when we are having a picture thought. They could read out body language for a change.

We definitely need to devote classes to picture conversion, where we could learn what about a picture was important. We could devote some energy in figuring out what really is normal in terms of picture thought development and blend our new knowledge into new education standards. We would learn to use aids like hearing filters and pressure devises to cut down on our overload and conversely little tricks to pre think Autistic situations so that faster thought might be possible. We would need to spend a lot of time on movement and motion. Walking talking and chewing gum are not easy for someone autistic, and if get used to doing that stuff and getting used to the noise that goes with some of that stuff it would make us more able to handle task in later life, like driving. We might even start kids of on bikes and then move on to rowing to develop (sense of motion and teamwork) more senses. We might even drive golf carts as the ultimate experience. By doing this stuff correctly we would develop a better sense of when and how to turn our Autistic thought off and on. Driving would be a breeze if our supersenses were already adjusted for it and we learned not to think in pictures while driving.

Even if all of this advise is totally wrong it might be more right than the current MR/DD thinking. At least we had lots of success on our own. Frankly I feel the modern Autisitc has been cheated (not on purpose) by an education system to bogged down to count its own toes. Our own "Experts" have not been a lot of help especially subscribing to the MR/DD bandwagon. Time, forbid I hope we never experience another Sing-a-Long or loud echo filled classroom! I think there are a lot good ideas that came from modern Autism that need to be carried on but even the best of things will not work in a loud noisy school. Perhaps, Someday we will not be forced to endure lots of eye contact that traditional thinkers claim we need. We will really done our job well if someday others can actually read our body language and tell when we are done with a thought. Don't worry some day the eye contact will come as will social charm but when we are young and learning Picture Thought we need to be able look at our developing thoughts. You would never keep the number line away from view of a traditional thinker, so our blank stare is like us looking at a number line. When we finally learn the many versions and combinations of Picture Thoughts We will use Picture-in-picture to look at you and also think Autistically. You will finally get the eye contact then.

A word about Experts, First off—I am not one—I am just a 'lucky devil' that happened to figure out there are two different things going on in Autism. For the most part Autism is gross ignorance. If anyone likes any of these ideas and want to borrow them build on them, improve them, they have my blessing. But please don't elect yourself "Chief Expert". Let time be the judge of that. Autism has had more than its share of them in its time.

Autism a Thing of the Past?

I know there are a lot of theories of where Autism came from, ranging from modern causes like a vaccination to a birth condition, to you name it. Well, maybe Autism is rooted in the past in earlier editions of man. PBS and National Geographic and Discovery Channel Viewers, as well as, people of science know very well the evolution of man theory. We have the skeletons. One can only assume they had a different thought process than ours but yet who knew how they were thinking? We have yet to discover their brains, or for that matter understand our own.

Autism might simply be an earlier version of man's brain. There is so much of Autism that fits well into a primitive life. Assuming this is true and possibly we descended from animals, the Autistic super hearing would be perfect. If I were Fred Flintstone (cave man cartoon character) or his earlier cousin I would expect to be able to hear like a dog. That high-pitched stuff could easily save my life or give me a head start, when being chased.

Feelings that are oversensitive today might have been just right if the body was covered with hair and one was basically naked. The "immunity" we have to the cold would have been great. The lack of pain feeling would have been handy, as there was not a medicine cabinet or a chemist in sight. The body can do a lot to heal itself if one could tolerate the pain or in our case even feel it to begin with. Like primitive man could have ever gone to the ER anyway? Well, at least modern Autistics can go to the ER but most of the time is a wasted trip as we break the first rule of medical etiquette We don't feel pain. If we don't feel pain how can we be hurt?

Most importantly however is picture thought. There was no one to speak to; no language to, no road maps and Fred's cousin would have been well served with a photo-based mind, like Autism. The Picture based Mind could easily make its own connections, draw its own maps that would tell where home was or the direction of a certain cave. Autistic thought could told the person in a Picture-in Picture thought or a Motion Picture thought how to prepare a killed animal or how to use a certain tool. Smell could have easily triggered picture thoughts, just like the do today. Over time (1000's of years) words could have been added and eventually became more dominant in survival and the Autistic part of the brain might have changed roles. We know today a few missing genetic items in a person's make-up and there is a good possibility of all kinds of trouble like Downs Syndrome, MS and Cerebral Palsy. Maybe there is just such a marker for Autism?

So now we have a new born baby that might have indeed been Autistic since birth or possibly a baby with a series of birth defects and conditions or injuries or one of a thousands of other factors that can't think normally. Did Mother Nature simply go back to plan "B" figuring some thought was better than none at all? Or did the Autistic ever start off normal? Were we miswired from the start? Maybe certain connections were never made to match the brain to evolution. Maybe Autistics don't even use left and right sides of the brain.

Sadly and I mean sadly, normal people in the last 100 years or so were given too much power at once and now we think were god herself. Normal is now whatever or whoever screams the loudest no matter if they are right or wrong. Traditional people can not as a rule be challenged with out an emotional irrational fight. They typically tend to hate first (very Primitive) naturally, and eventually learn to love others. Normal people are instantly correct and so inflexible that all-odd thought and ideas are simply ignored, we are the 'know it all's' our parents warned us about when we were teenagers. Don't forget it has been less than 100 years since the psychology we treat as "gold" came into being and medicine itself fell into modern times by accident along with it. In the millisecond blip of modern times it is still very likely that there are good chances Autistic brains are still genetically possible. Just think if the Autistic brains were figured out it might help pinpoint and cure other mental illness types of problems. Maybe they to are related to a Primitive Brain?

Yes, were flying around the globe in primitive riveted together buckets of aluminum with rockets strapped to them, and we have been to the moon and back and we can even tell where standing with in a foot or two anyplace on earth, but were still lost in a lot of respects. Most of the invention and discovery of modern times was bound to happen just since they were firsts of an era. If Ford didn't put the world on wheels someone else would have. It was only in the late 1940's that Autism was discovered, and in the 1970's that it was prematurely developed before and in between then Autism's quiet success was simply deemed insufficient and not worth a second look. I hope we just got done taking two steps backwards and there is a leap forward soon to come.

7

The Obsession Automotive Progress in the Works

No book on Autism would be complete with out a section dealing with the primary interest of the writer. Temple had her special knowledge on all the aspects of cattle, my specialties are automobiles and things mechanical. As you gathered from reading this far Mechanical Splinter skills have been both my curse and blessing. My first job working on cars was at a local Cadillac dealership and some of the bigger events follow. I love to hear about the obsession of other Autistics, total dedication to something brings out the best in everything and solves many problems.

I had worked for the Cadillac dealer for nearly a year and was still unaware of my Autism. But I was acutely aware I had a special "gift" of simply knowing what to do to fix a car. Although, I had the answer or at least the course charted to find the trouble my ideas seemed so strange and out of place that if they were given any thought at all it was usually ignored. I had a deep realization that my co workers 'top professionals' in car repair were painfully ignorant of the cars they were working on, as every mechanic has been since the days of the Model "T". Even Henry Ford didn't understand the car he had built: if he did the carburetor would have been invented along with the motor not after it. Henry's first car had a simple pipe gasoline was just poured in to. He had a hard time making it run. Henry it seems was just tinkering and happened upon his success as did many others in the early days of the automobile. There were a lot of firsts to discover in those days.

I soon found at the Cadillac garage that I was doing my repairs on my own, and they were working. One our best customers had just purchased a beautiful black Cadillac Seville with all the options including the top of the line radio system that played a song all its own whenever it was operating. The hum was understandably driving the customer crazy. I realized instantly when I moved this car around the shop and played with the radio, that the problem was in the speakers. When I adjusted the controls to play one speaker at a time I realized the hum was nearly gone when the R Rear speaker was turned off. Looking in the trunk the trim screw through the wiring harness was obvious. This logical approach, of finding the common factor, or reducing the problem to its smallest element allows for great troubleshooting. Also, required in this approach is the uncommon knowledge of what is really happening within the motor and its sub-systems: realization of electric and vacuum functions are also a big key.

At this point in my employment I had the reputation of being strange as well as Gay. The top mechanics were assigned to the car and soon parts were being replaced left and right. The radio was sent off to the repair shop and it was returned not surprisingly, to me at least, marked "OK," nothing wrong with it. The mechanics stewed over the return of the radio for several lunch breaks complaining the radio shop was surely mistaken. It was sent out again and once more it was returned. In an attempt to repair the hum aftermarket noise suppressors were soon hanging like Christmas ornaments on a tree connected to about every electrical thing on the car, the hum, although quieter, was still there. Meanwhile the owner was getting second thoughts on his purchase and was threatening to request his money back. The owner of the dealership was frantic and soon requested we call in the G.M. troubleshooter. She was here, gone and done in a half-an-hour and as the chief mechanic recalled for many lunch breaks to come, she barked, "Fix that wiring harness!"

He actually had said many more un-repeatable comments than that; she was a person of color after all, and worse yet she knew her stuff better than he did, talk about a hurt ego? The screw was removed from the harness and the radio instantly became quiet. Imagine that! If I had been on easier terms with Autism and the people at work as well, I'd fixed the radio on the Monday it came in. I had an urge to be militant so to speak as form of protest, it seems my coworkers always discounted my ideas. This was my way of getting even. Funny it seems I learned that behavior after I learned the 'normal emotions' like those around me. I really think, if I were handle that situation correctly, by fixing the car and relating it to the people in charge I'd needed the equivalent to an ambassador. I really hated to "just" fix the car on my own as the part replacers would have simply assumed one of their fixes would had done it. Today years later I have figured out enough socially to effectively tell someone the story to go along with the strange idea.

In another instance another Cadillac had been in the shop for seemingly months on end with a stalling problem. Our top mechanic had replaced about every part imaginable and still the car would stall. He was even replacing parts that were not even common to all cylinders. I realized when I drove this car the steering was binding, I could hear it in the wine of the power steering pump that didn't match the sound (another trouble shooting advantage) of all the other Cadilliac's I'd driven. When I inspected under the hood, I had seen the Steering Gear adjustment screw was off, turned in a thread too far, it had to be too tight. I made arrangements on the sly to return the car to the customer's house and on the way I stopped off in a drug store parking lot and loosened the adjustment and suddenly the car ran fine. The overtightened gear was really too much strain on the motor. Granted a tight gear was expected in a new car, but these pathetic motors in the Cadillac of this era were lucky to run at all when all systems were working correctly; if anything was askew, forget it. The problem must have been solved, as she never returned for that problem.

LUELLA *my child my life*

If I wasn't the odd one at work I was for sure the odd one at home. I had set out on fixing the rusted out frame on our family owned since new 62 Pontiac. Luella, as she is known is the first car I'd ever drove or cared for was "family "to me just like a spouse might be. Yes, maybe it is a case of that strange Autistic attraction to objects rather than to people but never the less I had to save Luella from the junkyard more than one time. I had saved her by protesting loudly every time the idea of junking the old car was brought up. Eventually everyone was so tired of my protesting they finally gave up and kept her.

Perhaps Luella is THE WORST car General Motors ever made, it stands to reason. She was the third best selling car in 1962 but yet few of them survive. Ohio my home state has less than 100 of them registered. The pictures taken in of the junkyard s in the late 1960's help explain that as most were there due to rusted out frames. More of them survive in dryer climates but if rust didn't take them the badly designed engine rocker arms killed the motors. If all else failed the Slim Jim transmission, a cheap cost cutting measure certainly fell apart probably about the same time the frame was discovered to be rusted out.

Luella and I drove each other back and forth to school and many times and I even walked home, a few times, as she'd quit running again and again. Throughout the two years I drove her to school she was towed no less than 18 times, all for the same problem,' Fuel pump'. I discovered on what would have been the 19 episode that it actually ran setting on the step hill that she had quit on this time. My auto career was born right then and there when I realized the 'fuel pump' had never been the trouble, the tank outlet had been plugged all along. With that experience, I made a commitment to my self to be become the best automechanic possible.

Luella has had her share of troubles besides the fuel system and a rusted out frame. Just after I'd started driving her only a few weeks after getting my licence I also discovered how to descend steep hills with no brakes! I was pulling into the school parking lot and 3/4 of the way down the steep hill that formed the entrance to the school the brakes failed. Surprisingly, I didn't panic I simply drove in circles in the thankfully somewhat empty parking lot to 'rub off' some speed. I don't think Autistics can think fast enough or far enough ahead to panic. Rather I simply figured out how I was going to cross a busy street into another lot, as the people driving in to this lot from the other direction were unaware I had no brakes and I wasn't simply "drunk". Finally across the street I finally thought to use the parking brake and brought Luella to a stop with two tires over the curb headed into a creek.

Soon I was surrounded by students and teachers that had seen the event and heard the motor screaming motor as I flew off the hill, and through the parking lot. I think they were asking if I was all right, and commenting, "Good driving" etc. I hope I wasn't to cold to the kindhearted people and thus perceived as cold and crude, but honestly I was looking at the fenders to see if I'd bent them jumping the curb. It took me several hours to realize just what could have happened and how caring those people were. I never did tell dad more than the brakes went out. If he'd known of the whole story she'd been history.

Anyway after graduating high school I discovered while doing an oil change on Luella that her frame was really rusty just in front of both doors. By the time I quit pounding on the frame with a hammer: to see just how bad it was there was a big 4" hole all the way through on both sides of the frame. Really, that should have been the end of her. Poor dad, he didn't even wince when I announced plans to replace the frame. *In my Pictures I had it all figured out, the derrick I'd build to set the body on, And just how I'd pull the frame, out from under it. It was the first time I'd built something that exactly matched my pictures.* I was so proud of my self.

Soon the body was setting in "mid air" atop the derrick and the frame was simply drug out from under the body. It would be eight years before dad could fully use his garage again. Between saving up money for the repairs, and not being satisfied with the repairs and discovering all the possible parts cars were in Arizona, it was quite a wait. I found out all 62 Pontiacs operated here in the rust belt (road salt in use in winter) were mechanical fodder due to a design flaw in the frame. I was showed a picture of a local junkyard taken in 1967 and it was filled to the rim with 61 and 62 Pontiacs all had rusted out frames. The operator told me this was the most of any one car he had ever had in his lot at one time, except for the Model 'T' after WWII.

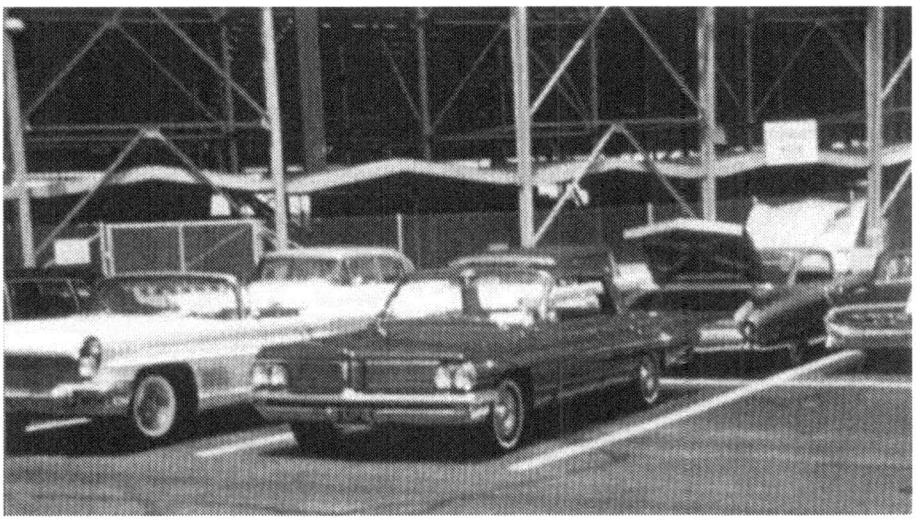

Luella, taken at the Lambda Car Club Grand invitational, Indianapolis Indiana. Indianapolis Speedway is in the background.

I'm proud to report today Luella is alive and well and in one piece, and we still travel together on occasion. Literally the day after she was completed and reassembled she proved her new found road abilities with a six hour after dark trip to Indianapolis Indiana for Lambda Car Clubs Grand Invitational being held there that year. Except for a minor repair, and some strange noises coming from the transmission about Dayton Ohio she performed very well. The noise was instantly, Autistically diagnosed as a leaking accumulator valve. *My picture thoughts assured me this was nothing serious as I watched the valve operate in relation to the noise I was hearing. (YES while I was driving) Figuring the hydraulic circuit of the transmission I confirmed my pictures by shifting manually via the gear shift and eliminating the need for the Accumulateor function and she was quiet.* The picture thought showed the computer animation of her transmission running both mechanically and another similar pictures showed the hydraulic circuit. Anyone else would have had to look a service manual to see the same pictures. By the time she made it back home the transmission seals had expanded enough for correct quiet operation. Really, only an obsessed Autistic would sweat all those details to keep a 'friend' in the family. I hadn't learned my lesion yet.

Building a Performance Car.

Along the way I also developed an attraction to a 79 Mecury Cougar that was a hand me down from other family members. Big Merc as she was known became the automotive experiment of all time. For the last 4 years she has stopped with the aid of a custom designed and built by myself Four-wheel-disc brake system. If only I could get Merc to start as fast as it stops I' have a Porchse. Merc is so much an obsession but it was more of a challenge. Again I had a point to prove of my mechanical abilities, but again I'd needed a diplomat to convince anyone but the closest family member of my plans and the confidence I had in them.

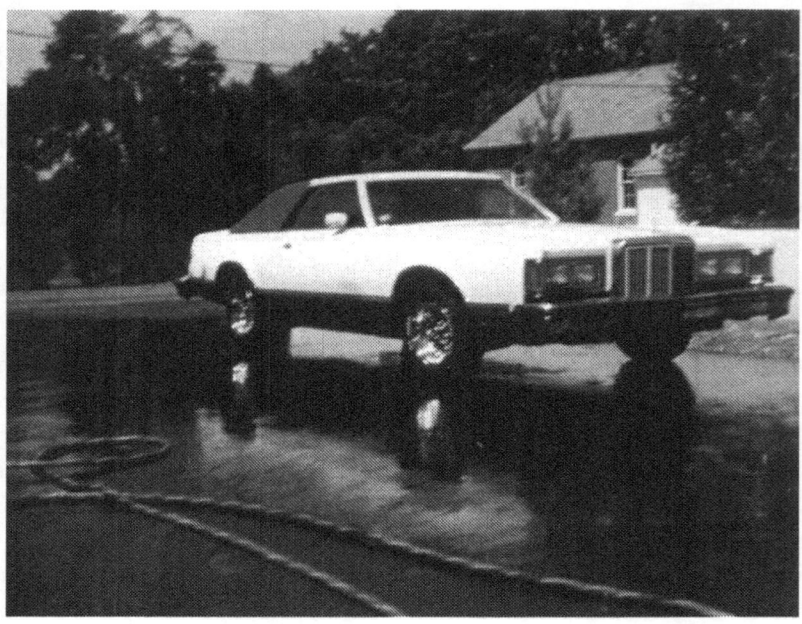

"Big Merc" taken years after her brakes were re designed.

Merc's rear brakes had failed, due to a design flaw relating to weak materials used in some of the major braking components. I found that the broken parts were no longer available, from Ford or even Bendix the manufacturer. The fixed, translated re-welded parts were proving to be worthless, as the weld would break again, after a short time. This car was too big for only two working front brakes. Not being able to afford a new car (used) I decided to revise Merc partly as a challenge and mostly out of necessity.

I went to the library and studied the Hollander Interchange Manuals, a set of books that tell what parts interchange with-in the different cars and even among the different brands of cars. I found no official interchange for any of the brake parts I was seeking but I was interested when I seen a 'special' Ford axle with rear Disc brakes. I found an example of that axle in a local junkyard mounted on a Lincoln Mark V and spent some considerable time measuring it up. Autistically, *I set and studied the axle, all of its details including the angles of the supports the lengths of the axle tube etc. using still pictures. I used the "laser" beam part of my thoughts to do the measurements. I used motion pictures to view a working model of the axle including the conditions of the car in a hard turn and fully loaded and how that would effect the axle and the stuff mounted on it. I used my pictures to design and build the brackets I would need to build it, to make it work and the routing of the brake lines and hoses. All of this was done setting in the junkyard!* And I couldn't pass Algebra?

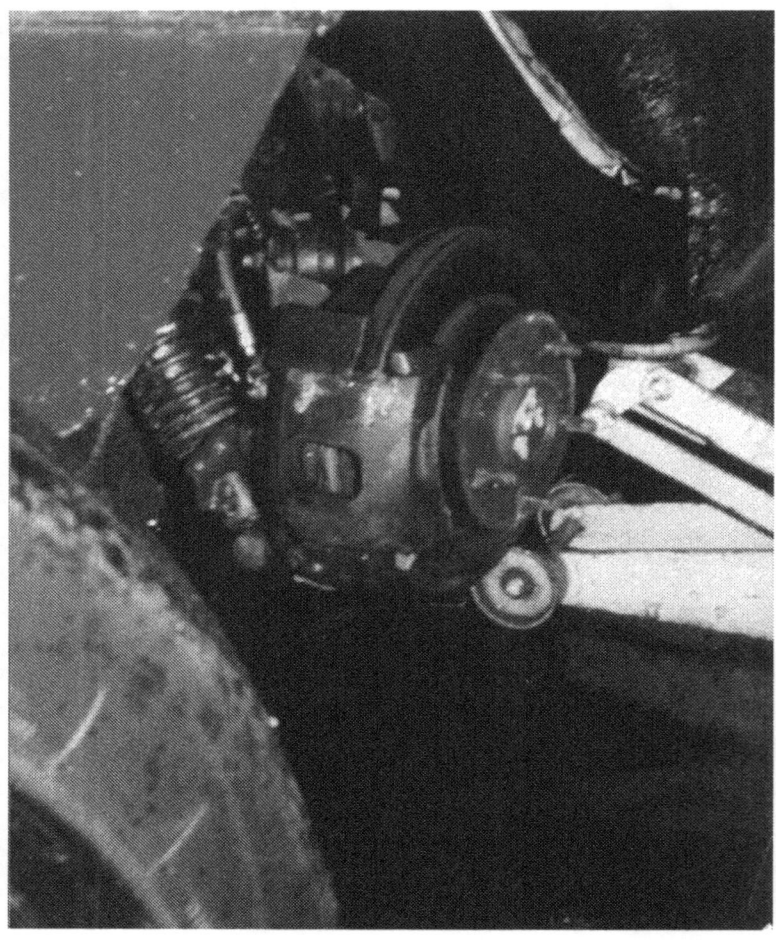

This was like one of my several 100 engineering pictures I had setting in the junkyard.

I autistically made the mistake of telling the junkyard employees, what I intended on doing with the axle and they were all torqued up over the idea. "That interchange was not listed in their manuals", they screamed and nearly didn't sell it to me. It took a heated discussion on my part to convince them to let it go. In some respect I was proud of my self for figuring out just how this axle was going to work, that I felt a need to drop the hint. I always felt a need to show up the parts replacers masquerading as mechanics but with out a Public relations firm, on my side I made many Autistic blunders. I now know I should have kept my mouth shut and simply drove the finished product to their door. Once home I realized all my calculations were correct thus the job would go as predicted.

I had started to install this axle and in its preparation I had stood it up on its end to let the old dirty oil drain from its axle tube. What a Mistake that was! *Soon the axle was falling and about to hit the concrete garage floor and my Pictures showed the potential stress fracture on the axle tube when it would have hit the floor, and the heated debate I had with the junkyard employees. The next thing I knew I was holding the entire axle assembly in my arms inches from the ground.* **That was the first time in my life I ever screamed in pain!** It took me ½ hour to stand up again. With only some minor pain, (for me at least) I was busy installing the axle under the car. It was a full month later before I ended up in the E.R. sicker than I'd ever been in my life. Normal people would have been in the hospital instantly. Of course as your aware as of this writing were still dealing with the effects of this injury. (I still hadn't heard of Autism yet!)

Despite the **_INJURIES_** and the simple building and engineering challenges, The thrill of Merc's first stop was unbelievable it was like shifting into reverse! All of the engineering and workmanship has proven faultless over the last 50 thousand miles. I even super tested it by towing and stopping three farm wagons of straw with it going down hill; it felt like nothing was back there! I drove Merc for years after wards and was delighted beyond belief with every stop and even once a week of so done a hard stop or two just feel the de-acceleration. The only design change to the original plan was the addition rear disc brake coolers (air ducts) to cool the rear brakes. In reality it wasn't necessary but better performance could be obtained if the brakes were cooled with the air flowing under the car. It was interesting to note the coolers proved to be really effective and driving on a dirt road, one could see in the mirrors the dust flowing from the rear wheels, proving the air dams worked.

Over the year Merc's other problems have required the invention/addition of electric cooling fans as the original belt driven one proved to be a killer as bit and pieces of it broke away, or if your really "Lucky" entire blades broke away. In fact many mechanics were injured while working on these car with the hood up and the motor running as the blades broke off. Of course, the picture thought engineering had this problem figured out in a few short thoughts. Besides never being able to keep a water pump on the car, Since the fan was out of balance, the "WILLIOW-Wish" sound of the fan spinning (autistic hearing) told me the fan was ready to fall apart. Again I was in the junkyard my version of Walmart collecting the parts I'd need and within the day I had two relay controlled electric fans installed. One would have been sufficient but I figured two might better in case one broke. If I ran both at once I could actually see the coolant gauge drop setting still at idle. Merc sounded like a vacuum cleaner when those fans were running.

To keep the tired old motor running I designed and installed an electric vacuum pump that in effect is CPR. The pump operates automatically as needed and simply supplies vacuum to the motor as the motor is no longer able to produce enough on its own. Again motors are nothing more than vacuum pumps. Think of it as cross between a supercharger and a turbo charger only it works better. Most normal mechanics would have replaced the carburetor in an effort to make it run but, I never found it necessary to replace a carburetor nor have the one or two other engineers I have spoke with that really deeply understand the motor. Merc still runs fine on her original at 210,000 miles. I really confuse the typical mechanic when I talk of vacuum the powerful but mostly invisible agent that makes the world work, Airplanes create vacuum over their wings to make them fly, T.V. tubes need it as well as many other things. Maybe since the concept of vacuum is such an invisible process kind like Autistic pictures, it lends its self to my picture style thought.

I really enjoy working on today's 'high tech." cars I generally find if I fix the 'Model T' that hasn't changed all that much from the originals, the "high tech." is often of good enough quality to fix its self. In my opinion the average mechanic has never understood the model "T", so it is no surprise the computers scare him as well. I have a long and varied history of fixing the tough stuff, the stuff others run away from. I have a dream if all works out well physically: If I can get to the point I can walk with ease again I plan on opening my own diagnosis only repair shop. Trouble shooting of course would be the speciality. I might as well earn a living from this obsession.

Really, everyone Autistic needs an advertising firm behind them weather their speciality is music computers cooking electronics or whatever. The wonderful ideas we have tend to be light years ahead of normal thought. But, even the best ideas don't work if they're locked in. I was lucky and had the chance to experiment and prove my self in a calm understanding environment. That insight gleaned from experience proves that we have many abilities that are locked in side. I think that the normal mind that wastes so much brain power figuring out the social aspects of life like who is who and 'where' do I stand in the eyes of others has lost it's ability to really think about problem solving. If other Autistics think like me there normal state of mind is typically serious, serious, serious were always finding the solution to a problem but unknowingly creating a bigger one by not being able to communicate to our emotional counterparts. Some of that serious thought however, is busy processing information and dealing with creating the pictures we will need to think with. If the Autistic hasn't developed serious picture thought yet I suspect s/he might just be simply drawing a blank. Fun doesn't seem to be pre-programed in our minds. When we do have fun most people would consider it work.

Developing new motors setting new standards.

Other off shoots of this mechanical ability include a ceramic motored 2 cycle gasoline trimmer that I made by converting an off the shelf trimmer. I have been fascinated for years with ceramic motors and often read about them in the magazine Automotive Engineering at the library. Ceramic motors according to some schools of thought hold the potential for being super efficient and lightweight. It seems not many of them have been real dependable but mine on the other hand mine is 7 years old now and seems to just keep going. My motor started out as a common off the shelf motor and I bored out the cylinder and replaced the bored out material with a ceramic paste that I made and had fired. I then pressed the new cylinder into the motor and custom fitted the related parts.

After some wild unexpected first runs and teething troubles like flames streaming out the muffler and the motor running too fast too easily I made some more new parts to solve various troubles and it has been running great ever since. A few years back I took a job at a local cemetery just to have the opportunity to use it for hours at a time in an endurance test of sorts, and it performed very well. My goal in making the motor was more to find a suitable ceramic capable of with standing stress more than making or creating a super efficient motor.

Pushing the Model "T" Motor out of the dark ages.

Just imagine some big Sport Utility Vehicle (SUV) getting 40 miles per gallon and still having good towing power? Think of a smaller car getting 60–70 MPG and an economy car topping 100mpg. I might have developed the engine to do it. My Autistic reasoning and splinter skill engineering have been working on this problem for years and thus I have invented a new more efficient motor. It is a combination of many things and blended technologies and even features a catalyst in the combustion process all promising a possibly 70% efficiency rating.

Today's best and highest tech stuff despite the hype of the advertising department is still only 35% +/-only slightly improved over the 100 or so years since the Model "T" set the world in motion. Emissions promise to be low helping to make the world a bit greener as well.

The Idea of this motor is so radical and somewhat simple that it would probably be perceived as stupid in many engineering circles. It is just far enough removed from the current motors to be radical and the Engineers of the world probably take too much faith in their standard text book education's and comfortable jobs to think too hard on "changing a good thing". Of Course I WISH I could draw what my Picture thought sees. If I'd just be able to 'stamp my head on the table' and have the drawing appear on paper this wild somewhat unexplainable idea would make more sense to the average person. Just like everything else I've built I can build what my mind figures out, I'll have to do the same with this.

Another endeavor I have planned is the invention of a concert quality player piano system that can play one note or the entire piece, correctly. My motivation for this was year ago I met a concert pianist suffering from a debilitating condition that was severely affecting her playing, especially in one hand, and I thought what a joy it would be for her be able to play again. She was slowly being reduced from the likes of Bhrams to Chop Sticks.

This piano system would unitize a computer off stage to monitor the notes played against the prestored-programmed notes and in conjunction with 88 "actuators" hit the missed notes. Gleaning some ideas from the Model T of all things the actuators would be a combination of electric and vacuum plungers placed strategically out of site depending on the application. Fine accurate control of the notes being played would be possible thus it could be used in a concert quality environment.

These projects and many more are more than just work, their actually my life and sometimes entrainment. Literally using my picture thought I can visualize the complete the piano system working and even the stress forces being generated within the running trimmer motor. I can sit and engineer (remember the working computer animation model I spoke of earlier) or reengineer most anything. Sadly this type of odd thought isn't real conductive to more social types of thought, thus I'm having to learn the ways of the wild emotional type thinker, something the rest of the world takes for granted. It might just a big as chore for the emotional (normal thinker) to learn our Picture Process.

It Is the Carburetor!   *And other automotive myths.*

That saying has been around since the early days of automobile and is as false today as it was then. However the 98% of all mechanics believe it to be true, for whatever reason. With reasoning of that caliber it is obvious to me at least that correct car repair is totally an accident if the mechanic actually figures out a problem and better yet completes the repair with out making a bigger problem no matter if the car is high tech and 'modern' or a model with a few years on it. Most mechanics are as ignorant of their work as can be and like Autism there is a false sense of knowing all about it and being satisfied with that. Why else do we have 1000's of cars that can't be repaired, and even personalities like National Public Radio's, Car Talk Guys.

Some 100 years ago the first repair shops opened and ignorant mechanics were typically on equal footing with what they were working on. That means there were few parts to replace and a good guess was all that necessary to get something running again. That was the start of trouble and officially called the Flat Rate Repair System that is still used to this day. Basically it means the Mechanic gets paid for replacing parts and by the way for doing it as quickly as possible. Certain repair jobs like replacing a water pump for example might pay 1 ½ hours labor to the mechanic for replacing it. If the mechanic can do the job in ½ hour he still gets paid 1-½ hours. If the job takes longer or comes back it still pays 1-½ hours. Well, that is O.K. to a point but it provides no reason to actually learn and appreciate what is really going on inside the workings of a car. Thus we now have generation after generation of parts replacers and an entire industry based on the first primitive repairs of the model "T".

While the mechanic is in the shop turning tricks and playing beat the clock, methods used to improve his odds of doing that including power tools and the like help, but, they often make more trouble. When the flat rate guy strips out or cross threads a bolt using a power tool he often never knows the mistake. However the next person to work on the car often gets stuck repairing the previous repair and ultimately the customer pays for the repair. Air tools would never be allowed in my shop for assembly purposes, dis assembly would be acceptable. People mechanics included don't realize how fragile and close toleranced and yes cheap metal can be; it commands more respects than it gets. To make matters worse, often cheap cut rate parts are installed to help in the profit margins in some cases in my opinion there is little difference if the part is original GM. Ford or Chrysler, in fact the new part might actually be better than the original. However Toyota and other quality makes suffer from many after market parts.

Automobiles done correctly can be a pleasurable worthwhile experience. By done correctly one needs to start with a good basic design, well ok, a Toyota for example. I have sifted through junkyards and repaired all kinds of cars and autistically studied the in and outs and have found basic design makes all the difference. If only the Toyota mechanics were as good as the cars. Many better makes are over engineered well thought out and have many back up systems and typically have quality components. Then there is the rest of the fleet; a scary lot of haphazardly make it run engineering automobiles that often never overcome their shortcomings and reliability troubles. They were doomed from the start.

Imagine if I told you my own car has two drive shafts operating off the engine, the motor is center mounted and it has 200,000 miles on it and still worth a small fortune. It is true and it is a Toyota Previa mini-van. There is so much stuff on that van that GM Ford and Chrysler could never do like pump oil from a convenient reservoir to the center mounted motor. I'd be surprised if Gm could do that without a leak or mechanical fault or overfilling the motor. I wouldn't be shocked to see the lack of thought in their system. I'd be even more shocked to see two drive shafts running off the same motor, and for sure many other mini-vans have trouble just running. I just can't figure out why so many poor designs leave some manufacturers lines. I probably already own the worst car GM ever made my 62 Pontiac (according to the registrations only 3 % survive) I have personally dealt with Ht 4100 Cadillac motors from the early 1980's. It was called the hook and tow 4100,'highly troubled', a hand grenade all well defining names reflecting the obvious state of this poor motor. This motor typically required a new crankshaft or bearings every 30,000 miles and it took 5 minutes to check the oil as it took it that long for all the oil to drain back. I could co on and on Chrysler and Ford and yes-even Toyota all have had some lemons to their credit. Personally, I recommend <u>Consumer Reports</u> magazine when it comes time to buy new or used car. Their non-profit non-biased reports make the automotive experience much more bearable. Their reports include repair histories and real world testing. Buying their best improves your odds of getting a reliable car.

A word about rental cars as used cars

I would guess a lot of used cars started out life as a rental car and while that is not all bad some of the rentals I have experienced have been through hell. Working in the industry, I have seen them idle for hours at a time and even idle through a complete tank of full gas. I have seen them get so cold on a 90' f day that that frost formed inside the car and even lowered the temp of engine compartment substantially as the air conditioner iced up. I have seen the oil added only when the oil light flickered or the motor knocked. 5000-mile oil changes are the norm and many were even beyond that. In my years in the business I have lost count how many I have seen go through he car wash with the fuel tank door open and gas cap off. The employees did this poor treatment; the customers did their share of damage as well.

I guess there is something about the idea it is not my car, as the customer drives it a bit rougher than necessary. Then there is the lost syndrome where the customer renting it is in a strange town in a strange car and suddenly decides it is necessary to jump a few curbs or something else just as stupid to make an exit or a turn. The car is in effect dropped kicked. To add to the trouble many employees are first time drivers and the cars get a little more abuse from their careless mistakes. NOT ALL of the cars have been through this type of hell but, there is hardly any way to tell until you own it and might be grief stricken with problems. As with the purchase of any used car, one must be careful and if you suspect it might have been a rental look it over really carefully and reject it if has the smallest of problems.

Trouble Shooting

Well, it helps if you understand every thing going on in the car: it is easy. My self included I know of 5–6 mechanics worldwide that truly understand what is going on in a motor and subsystems of a car. Most mechanics are good parts replacers and very honest. Sometimes, no matter how hard a mechanic tries circumstances conspire against him or her and make them appear to be dishonest. Also sometimes plain old ignorance contributes to unnecessary or poorly performed repairs that sometimes reflect poorly on the mechanic. It is also true that many mechanics are really not trained nor have educations beyond high school. Sadly, the people working on your are not only ignorant of the Model "T" they are totally ignorant of the computers and high tech items and pollution control devises. Thankfully many mechanics are saved with the self-diagnosing features of today's computer driven automobiles. The self diagnose feature is guide and contrary to popular belief very limited as to what it can tell the technician. There are so many functions of a motor the computer does not monitor; thus it is impossible for the computer to 'know it all'. It seems ironic that over 80% of the engine is still splashed oiled just like the old 'T' motor it is based on was. Still it is called "High Tech"? As I have always said fix the model 'T' and the high tech will care for itself. Other things like logic also help, Is the problem common to all cylinders? If so why worry about parts not relating all cylinders.

Like it or not 'the high tech' is here to stay, it is the job of the computer to ensure the most efficient running of the motor and other systems. To hear the advertising department tell about the computer, it is for the good running of the car but in reality is just a benefit to having to manage pollution controls to meet strict clean air standards. Otherwise it is a safe bet the high tech would be left off if the manufacturers could live with out it. It is interesting to read some service manuals and discover the same car operated in Canada for example are often void of our computers and pollution control devices. (Used to be quite a regular occurrence)

Here is an another 'pet problem' of mine: motor oil. It is by far the most misunderstood and confused item when it comes to the car. Oil's last job is lubrication not its first as it is claimed to be. Due the design of the *modern motor* that is just the same as the model "T" Oil's first job is compression sealant. The oil splashes up around the pistons and seals the combustion. That is why oil turns black and gets dirty it collects the dirt from combustion. This is perhaps the one vital reason never to run your car low on oil it makes for more engine wear. After it has collected the dirt oils next job is the primary engine heater or cooler. Then it disperses and holds the dirt and finally is forced through the internal workings, the 20%of the motor that is pressure oiled. The other 80% of the motor is splash oiled. The oil filter gets the "rocks" but the "fine" dirt that eventually deposits itself on the inside of the motor causing poor performance, oil leaks and a "slow running" motor and sticky valves among other problems are the things that often confuse the average mechanic (and even computer systems) into thinking there is really trouble and in reality the motor is simply plugged up. If your experiencing a poor running car try changing the oil every 500 miles until it comes out clean and spotless at the 500 mile change. You be amazed what in 'effect' cleaning the dirt out of the motor will do for its performance.

By the way I change my oil when it becomes deep brown, this color indicates the oil is has picked up and held nearly all of the dirt it can hold and by the time it is black it is depositing the dirt it can not hold in the motor. The dirt simply attaches and deposits itself on everything making once easy moving parts in mobile. Valves no longer snap shut, the lifters start to stick sometimes-causing backfires and other troubles blamed on the computer. As for oil I use the cheapest oil possible that meets the API (American Petroleum Institute) classification I need. Even if I were a millionaire I would use the cheap oil. To get an API classification the oil is well tested and approved. Thus the oil for 99 cents a quart is just as good as the stuff for $2.00 a quart. Read your owner's manual to tell what class of oil you need, and buy the cheapest oil meeting the requirement. Also note the new trend toward 5 (light) weight oil is prompted more by the 5000 mile oil changes recommended by the manufacturers trying to get the car to hold together long enough to out last the warranty. In this case the 'thinner oil' is more likely to flow through the dirt that is bound to deposit at 5000-mile oil changes. I still like the idea of 10-weight oil changed when it gets deep brown. No, the computer has no way of knowing contrary to what the expert salesman or service person says of what type oil is being used and it makes no real difference most of the time.

Another Automotive Mystery

Vacuum *is the other part of the motor that is totally ignored forgotten and misunderstood. Smart Drag Racers in the 50's installed Vacuum pumps on the motors, it was cheap effective way to increase performance. The vacuum is typically what delivers the fuel (in carburetor equipped engines) and is also depelenished when the throttle is open. Eventually the motor runs so low on vacuum no more fuel can be sucked in. The vacuum pump simply keeps a higher vacuum in the motor allowing for faster acceleration.*

I bet there are a lot of mechanics today that don't even know what vacuum is about and there is such thing as ported and manifold vacuum produced by a motor. I have used vacuum to jump start engines by connecting a running motor to a non-running one via a vacuum hose. The vacuum hose is connected from the running car to the stalled one; it is in effect CPR for a tired motor. I also ran a car with out a working fuel pump my siphoning fuel from the fuel line with the vacuum (suction) from a vacuum hose. It was "weird" you stepped on the gas to slow down (open throttle and lowered vacuum (suction power)) and let up on the gas pedal **to** go faster.

Vacuum could be the most important diagnosing tool in engine repair but like many things miss-understood it is ignored. In some ways however it is not: automobile many computer calculations rely on vacuum readings. It seems at least to me, some engineer somewhere understands vacuum.

As Seen on TV

I get no more entertainment and aggravation than listening to an infromerical dealing with something automotive. I really get a kick out of the one where the air flow device is place in the air intake and "suddenly" the gas mileage goes way up? If the devise worked the factory would have installed it and what difference does it make how the air flows when entering the motor. If the Air pressure is 14,7 lbs. per sq. inch as average the right amount of air will be there for combustion. In fact until someone can change the efficiency of the combustion process not much can change otherwise. You can twirl the air all you want but only so much gets in the motor anyway.

Then there are magnets you place in or around the fuel system that again "help the mileage" then there is the "super oil" that kind of works only because it is so slippery. Long term use makes no account for the combustion dirt entering the oil thus the dirt is simply ground in to the "soft motor". Long term use of the super oil is probably less than 6 months for most cars, that is when something major will break with the use of that oil. Thankfully in this day and age of fuel injection the miracle 100-MPG carburetor are gone and again if that stuff ever worked the automakers would have done it. Again the efficiency of the motor is still low around 35%—that is the true limit to the mpg.

The miracle waxes and polishes make up another segment of the car care market and I'd guess most are only so-so at doing what they claim. I have seen decal inside windows declaring "protected by such-in-such product" and the paint is totally pealed off the car. Of course, that might be a manufacturer problem but if the protection was worth anything one would at least expect better results. When I worked for car dealer ships I often was not impressed with the stuff they push either. In fact the rust proofing was so bad that it needed to be touched up annually and also we took that opportunity to wash inside the lower doors (road salt and dirt collects there) and wash the under side of the car paying special attention to the inside the fenders. Even the worst of modern cars will remain rust free even operating in areas where road salt is used if it is washed properly Typically I try wash my car once a week and with a mild soap mixed with (Pam) and dry it with a back-back blower. The air dry leaves a spotless finish and even dries out around and under ornaments and trim on the car. My idea of rust proofing is Marine paint sprayed on the bottom of a new car. This Paint is meant to be under salt water—it is well suited to a car. Simply spray the bottom of the car with a garden sprinkler occasionally and you're set. We have done this trick for years now and none of our salt-subjected winter driving has affected our cars.

8

Misfortunate Listening

I have been cursed throughout my life, with many things but nothing more two sided than appearing and acting normal. While I should be thankful I can pull off the "trick" of being normal and being treated like one of the guys, the responsibility that goes with it is troublesome. Due to the slow motion thinking process; the translating and the processing and conversion of thought to speech, I often come off as the world's best listener. Sometimes all that entails is being host to the conversation of a person that is more than thrilled to tell you (or anyone that will listen) their take on things. Worse yet when I'm lagging behind their words and looking at them intently trying to get the gist of their speech, they get the impression that I'm really taking in all of their ideas. In reality, I have got an education on just how lonely and insecure many people are.

In other more serious matters I have been put into the role of Psychologist/Counselor and I'm so regretful of the outcomes. If I had known I was Autistic I realized that the people coming to me for advice and assistance were being unknowingly ignored by me I'd steered them to a better counselor. Both Mike a Co-worker and John a relative came to seeking advise on how to deal with the Gay Issue facing both of them. Both thought since I was "out" I'd be the perfect person to come out to, and get advice from. Granted I'm a good listener on the surface at least but no one realized I was missing the real clues being presented. In my learned social behavior I figured how to say 'oh that's nice' and similar phrases at key times and look at the party I'm talking with, many times I'm looking at thought pictures and not seeing them. I've learned to figure and predict where the conversation is going in an effort to keep up with it and in these cases where serious consequences were at stake the guessing at the meaning of my typical conversation was insufficient.

The reality never hit me until I was standing in front of Mike's casket in the funeral parlor. He was Gay! During our talks at work (we worked in the same department) I'd often get side tracked when I broke off the conversation while I waited on a customer, and then resume later where we had left off. During these conversations he was beating around the bush trying to tell me he was gay by mentioning San Francisco, his strict catholic upbringing and his strained home life. He was probably in hopes that I'd bring the subject of Gay up. I was 'out' but in the closet at the time, but I didn't openly talk about it at work. We even had some "guy talk" on some pretty personal stuff. But still he never said he was gay and, Autistic me—I never figured it out. I guess it would had to be painfully obvious before it sunk in. These days my Gaydar works really well, Gaydar is that sense of knowing, through experience that anther person is gay.

After our talks I was bugged by some of the phrases he used and still I never associated them with the danger he was in. I really had terrible thoughts the day I heard he was missing and had "stole" his dad's van and no one knew where he was. After work I set in the car trying to figure what was going on my picture thoughts kept going blank (was that emotion?) and I'd cry for a bit. I had to set there for twenty minutes before I had enough composure to drive home. The next day I heard the terrible news that he killed himself just as the a Police office pulled him over in Florida. Terrible to say I wasn't all that upset, it was over what is there to do. Every one else was in tears and flowing with emotion but autistically it never really sunk in.

His "girlfriend" cornered me a few days after the funeral at work and told me they had sent him to me for advice! That's great If only I'd known. I really felt bad now. Learning from this I really wonder if the conversation was reversed could some one Autistic communicate to others he or she might be in dire straights over a problem such as this? At this point my Autism discovery was still 10 years away.

Not quite a year after Mike's passing I met for the first time a step cousin John. John had enlisted in the Marines and was just out of high school. Little did I realize he was doing that (joining-up) to prove a point; that being he 'wasn't Gay.' Being out for some time now, I realize that is one "show" many people put on to prove to the world they are not gay or Lesbian. Play Straight. In Fact many Gay bashings are instigated by closeted Gay people. What better way to prove to the world you are not Gay?

John and I had met while we were working on his car after it had quit running and he was stranded at his Grandfathers house. (His grandfather, an X-Marine).

While we were working on Johns car he to brought up the Gay subject after a long hide and seek conversation and I was in the worst possible position to listen Autistically speaking, as I was deep in greasy motor parts and my thought pictures were frantic with mechanical thoughts and John was talking of personal thoughts. Finally during a break when I actually was having some conversation-related thoughts, he asked, "Are you "Out" to "Grandpa"? Without thinking I instantly commented, are you kidding? That would be the last person I'd ever come out to. The energetic hope and enthusiasm experienced by a teenager simply vanished and the look on his face was so "telling to me". Remembering Mike's funeral I spent the rest of our day's together trying to right my wrong and tell him he was OK and Gay is really normal for some of the population. I thought my message and hit home, as he seemed a lot more comfortable with Gay and even joked about it. Several months after boot camp he took his own life.

I wonder if the circumstances of the conversations were different and we were talking in a quiet non-interupted environment (in both situations) if I would have got the point they were both trying so desperately trying to tell me. I had just come to my own reality of Gayness so I should really been attuned to their similar situation. Still I was lost in my Autistic thoughts. As a child one of my biggest troubles, that still haunts me even today as you just read, with reading and communication was that it was "your" language and it seemed so illogical. Every word was a sound (and in our case) a meaning to itself. The "F" sound…and the "PH" sound were the same? Then why wasn't FAN spelled PHAN? What was so special about A, E, I, O&U, I tried figuring that one out for months, they were simply letters to me. An Autistic language might really be "precise and two the point", much like German. English is a romantic language and thus there is a lot more to learn about it I remember being overwhelmed with all of the different words that mean the "same" thing "2"=to, too and two, why not just "2"? I really thought when I overheard a group of mothers talking of the "Terrible 2's" they were referring to speech, and not the habits of a two year old.

I believe most moderately functioning Autistic school children will eventually figure out how to read and communicate, But, It will take longer than average. You'll find if the progress "follows" my example, it will be fast and sudden after a period of "hopelessness"—just when you thought you were going to give-up. Until the progress is demonstrated however, don't quit pushing the lesions and the exercises or they might get the idea whatever it is might not be important. Of Course if the Autistic could be taught in his native language—Pictures, learning would be quicker and once something was learned, effort could be made to convert it to normal thought.

As for pictures in a younger Autistic, I don't know if he would be having them yet? He might be seeing little "Blank black spots" at this point that 'if you will' might be considered "baby thoughts" My little blank thoughts were prevalent through out most of second grade. Then they became little color spots that I feel were undeveloped pictures. This may explain why an Autistic child might give the impression that he is drifting off, or not paying attention, but if he was like me he is really trying to figure out what was just said. IF YOU COMMUNICATE TO THE AUTISTIC STUDENT his thoughts are different from yours and he needs to make you understand his thoughts. That for the moment will be the best education advice I can give. IF I had known those thoughts were special I'd been using them long before 8th grade. Even today, when I require deep picture based thoughts, my eyes may be open, but I may not see what is in front of me, rather I'm seeing my thought picture.

I feel I'm lucky in that 30% of my thoughts are with out pictures and dare I say "normal". Generally, they are the simpler ones and only complicated thoughts need pictures. One of the reasons I feel I think somewhat normal is the fact I ignored the pictures until eighth grade out of ignorance. This was in effect training in how to become a normal thinker. I feel I'd done better over all thinking in my natural mode in pictures and in the long run grade school would have been much more rewarding. I feel once an Autistic pictures develop and "function" correctly the student will be able to make short cuts to them and communicate with a bit more ease. Even as well as I get along I can't even keep up with really important speech and content. If you need to have a really important conversation with someone Autistic, please talk slowly and deliberately allowing time for processing and their direct answers. Don't force feed them answers. You might even have them explain to you just what the conversation was about, you might be shocked of some of the details that were missed. Remember he will have to learn the picture thought on his own, sadly there is not much a parent can do, except encourage him/her to do his best, the best he can.

Even doing my best, and I have been told time and again, I function very well I still miss a lot of the details of the conversations I have. Maybe we learn the language well enough to pass the English course but with our "eye's shut" looking at our pictures we really do miss the body language and the subtle clues that make the real communication possible. We know the mechanics of communication but the secret code to unlock its meaning isn't there. Even the spell checker in my Word 97 Program that I'm using to write this is confused. It hates the word Autistically, It's program often gives me the message *"missing that"* when it doesn't realize some of the words I'm using are being considered nouns.

More than anything else my day to day life is most hampered by the "poor listening" actually hearing it all, coupled with the picture processing and thought conversation process all tend to make communication a questionable chore. I have finally started to respect that aspect of my life for what it is and finally for the first time in years have been able to hold a job, a simple one. I drive cars to and from an airport for a Rental Agency and it is Autistically boring but yet my normal functioning mind is working at near capacity just doing this job. The 30% of my normal mind that I must make a living with are only able to do a job of this nature, but it provides some income at least. My Autistic mind is board and idle but in order to use it effectively I'd need the ultimate job probably working in my own shop. I feel so little at times going to work to a job such as this but I have tried higher functioning jobs and they usually end up in disaster when my picture thoughts cannot keep up with the real world.

9

Pain What is That?

Pain: What is that?—_The experiment continues, this aspect of Autism is really like science fiction. Please, don't treat it as such it is really serious! Your understanding of it might prevent a lot of pain and suffering for your loved one. Ironically it also show s how deficient medical science really is, as well as, the study of Autism._

Pain tolerance is the other unrealized aspect of Autism. Just as pictures never reach the point of everyday conversation, the lack of pain is similarly ignored. Once again it might fall under the realm of out of sight out of mind, both Autistically and from mom and dads point of view. I really cringe when I hear an Autistic parent stating, "He's never been hurt". I bet he has and NEVER realized it, it is possible for Autistic people to walk on broken bones, horrible sprains and worse and not even "know" it. One they don't realize the pain there in themselves and of grave concern to me is a "normal" physical exam given by a "normal "doctor in a" normal" fashion is indeed worthless to an Autistic. Ever hear of dead man walking? Were a version of it.

If I could have one wish I'd wish to feel pain in the normal way the rest of the population does. I'd live with the picture thought. For once I'd be able to avoid injury since I'd have Mother Nature's early warning system and thus doctor's visits might be closer to normal. A typical office visit is indeed the odd experience as the 1–10 pain scale is USELESS as the highest I ever felt is a 2. I found over the years my "2" is actually a normal person's "8". Now day's whenever I feel the first hint of pain or notice something different, I instantly pay attention to it. The deeper in my body the pain is the less I feel of it. If the doctor pushes and probes in a normal fashion I feel nothing. However, if the doctor gently rubs the surface of the skin I actually the best chance of feeling something, even something deep at times. Black and Blue marks are not common, the injuries and bumps the average person gets a black and blue mark from is mostly unnoticed in the Autistic. How many Medical Schools' have ever taught anything on dealing with Autistic patients?

I for one could give them a few pointers some years ago I had the misfortune of being in an industrial accident where a large heavy car axle fell down on me. It should have been an 911event but instead it was a common lump in life that I had got used to. In fact it was the first time in my life at the age of 34 that I ever screamed in pain! I couldn't move for close to 30 minutes **_BUT_** within the hour I was busy working with the same heavy axle lying on my back on a creeper not feeling anything really serious. Stuff felt odd but not serious. A few weeks later I was sicker than I'd been in my life and I was practically living in the E.R. I wouldn't get home more than a few hours before I was back again. I was still ignorant of Autism at this point, but this would turn out to be a learning adventure and yet another section of this Autism experiment.

As a result of the injuries I had a CAT scan performed, and in the end the results showed the results of some terrible injuries that I suffered five years prior to the scan. I had been walking on a shattered hip joint and also have a deformed Rib Cage and only in the last 2 years have I ever felt anything close to pain. Sadly nowadays I feel constant pain that is an entirely new experience for me. When my doctor confirmed the X-ray results he was amazed I didn't feel all that damage and was really amazed I could walk. He also suggested organ in the brain called the Thalamus is disconnected or mal-functioning. It is responsible for interpreting pain. Autistic's are probably using their Thalamus to think with! Probably the reason I was void of broken bones was being Autistically aware, something like being drunk, in my normal sate of being I didn't react quick enough to tense up my body. The fallen axle simply rolled over my body and since I was not tense the force that might have broken my leg and hip was spread out over a bigger area. I had enough damage, as it was thank you. This the similar concept to a drunk driver walking away from an accident mostly unhurt, a somehow relaxed body isn't nearly a prone to injuries as one that is tensed up. Interestingly the older I get the less back and blue marks I get, and I never had all that many when I was child. Occasionally my injured hip will appear black and blue today from the "inside" other wise the only time I get a black and blue mark at all is when blood is drawn, and then it is a small one. I wonder if Autistics as well as, not feeling pain don't show it in terms of black and blue marks?

Imagine! The doctor or nurse experiencing the only patient in his/her career that doesn't feel pain! Odds are the patient will be considered not injured, or faking the injury. It might be very likely the patient is suffering from a broken bone and unaware of it. Via comment from my Internet page I heard from a person who told of her daughters hurting wrist. This yearlong affliction was being treated as a "Sprain" turned out to be a broken wrist! The doctor didn't think X-ray's were initially necessary and the patient didn't show signs of pain bad enough to warrant them. I feel anytime an Autistic person is injured X-rays need to be done on the first visit.

Before I realized I was autistic, I had Knee sugary on a "squished" joint that was injured due to improper bicycling (riding in wrong gear). I never felt the pain when riding that would have told me to 'ease-up' nor afterwards when the knee was swelled so bad that it couldn't be bent, still it really didn't hurt. The doctor commented it was one of the worst knees he'd ever seen. The day of the operation I walked with "ease" out of the hospital. Three days later when I returned for a follow-up visit the doctor nearly fell over when I walked into his office without crutches or pain. In fact, he was amazed, I should have been too.

In other cases stuff skin deep is really the most obvious and readily felt. The "skin senses" seem to be over reactive. No, wool sweaters for me! But amazingly I can sprain an ankle, walk on it all day, and not realize it until I take my shoes off at the end of the day. The rare black and blue swollen ankle is visually obvious but I have to retrace the happenings of the day to figure out where it most likely happened. Black and blue marks in general tend to lighter than the normal persons and often there not even there at all.

Almost a month after the injury I finally made it to the emergency room for the 4–5 times in two weeks. Each time I went in I was suffering from shock. Test and theories failed to diagnose my problem, as I showed no pain reaction to the exams. Punching, poking and pulling, by the fleet of doctors and nurses couldn't determine the afflicted area. Their tests were predicted on the belief that I'd show reaction when the injured area was encountered. Eventually the condition got bad enough that the simple probe of a finger would make me want to throw-up. No, I could not feel the initial pain of the exam but on the trip home I'd get sick, It was delayed reaction. I never have felt or experienced the serious feeling of shock instantly, but I have dealt with it, well after the triggering event. It seems to be a delayed reaction. I wonder if part of our nervous system is disconnected or all of those pictures require so much brainpower that what brainpower or function designed to feel pain is being used in some other way?

Of course the picture thought has to play a part in this accident and here is that side of the story. I caught the falling automobile axle while—*I was busy looking at my thought pictures of how I was going to install this axle in my car,* I had the axle standing in a vertical position against the a wall draining oil out of it. As the axle started falling toward my feet I became aware my feet were directly in it's landing spot. I moved a little bit. *My (sudden) thought pictures showed the predicted crack in the axle housing had it hit the concrete, and further they showed the heated debate I had had the employees at the junkyard who nearly didn't sell me the axle as the interchange manual said what I was doing was not possible. (I knew it would work)* Next, I found my self-holding the entire axle assembly inches from the floor, and I was screaming in pain. That was the FIRST time in my life I had ever screamed in pain. I was doubled over in pain for a half-an-hour before I could straighten up again. Not your average walk in the park.

Amazingly, an hour later I was busy installing the same axle under the car and really I felt nothing, perhaps a few odd feelings but nothing "really serious." A month later Dad was taking me to the E.R., as I'd been hardly able to walk for days as well as, I'd been sick all night. After telling them of the story I was checked all over, checked for hernias and nothing was really found to be askew. I was told to contact my doctor. We had hardly made the 30-minute trip home from the hospital before I was sick again and hadn't been home more than a few hours before I was back in the E.R. Again, I was sent home. Finally after the 3–4 time I was kept in the hospital overnight and seemingly doctor after doctor and nurse examined and probed all to find nothing wrong except for a high temp.

After my overnight stay I felt good and I was released when my tempature dropped below one-hundred. Again I told to see my doctor and it was thought the aliment was my appendix. My doctor gave me the unwelcome news if it was my appendix; it would have to be treated with drugs first, as I didn't have insurance. I was placed on the most powerful anti-biotac on the market and was given refills on it. The Pharmacist told me on the 3 rd re-fill, that if the trouble was not improved by now I should go back to the hospital as this indeed was the most powerful drug on the market. I had to agree with her as I felt no better and was even feeling worse.

That night while looking at my self in the mirror after a shower, I seen for the first time a split down the middle of my lower chest. The split was almost 4" and it stung if I touched it. If the skin would have been broken I could have stuck my fingers right in. As it was I could reach in quite a ways. This prompts the feeling of shock eventually, but nothing instantly alerting me to TROUBLE. When my doctor examined the wounds, he to could stick his fingers in and I felt nothing to speak of. However, now if the exam was too rigorous I felt the need to throw-up. He didn't think that was the trouble at all, I knew I should have faked a scream during the exam. I tried several other doctors while I still had a savings account and soon I was walking with canes and crutches. I ended up wearing a back brace meant for heavy lifting and it wasn't for my back but rather, it was found that if I held my stomach tight I didn't get sick as quick and could again go the whole day without much hassle. However, if I lifted too much or did too much activity I was again sick with symptoms of shock. One of the last surgeons I seen had his fingers right in the "hernia" (split) and said I can't find it, he stated, "I can't fix what I can't see." Believe me I have heard that statement many times in the past few years. Technically, I'd be more correct in stating the hernia was a muscle wall tear as no other body parts are pinched in them that we know about.

Finally with some sweet-talking from my mom, and qualification for H-cap (hospital care assurance program (welfare)) we were able to convince a surgeon to fix the visible hernia. The doctor was hesitant (understandably) and even had me draw the hernia on my stomach right before the operation. The operation was a success and I was really feeling pretty good again. However, I was still in recovery when the bill collectors started calling and I was not at all thrilled with them, so as a result I went back to work too soon and broke the newly repaired hernia open again. I felt great after all and Dad couldn't convince me to wait it out a little longer. Besides that wouldn't have been me: I was always up and going.

Before the hernia operation was done I also had x-rays done on my hipbone pelvis region as ever since the accident my hips have hurt. They claimed all was allright I had no reason at that time to distrust the doctors. At this point I had never seen the X-rays. Today they "can't be found". If an Autistic person can feel something it must be bad. No one medically seems to pay attention to that claiming that my hips "can't hurt there." Oh. Really?

I was back to where I was before in a matter of hours after the "hernia" busted. I could hardly stand or walk. I ended up wearing two back braces at once and by doing that I could stand and walk. Although the pressure felt good as Autistics like pressure devices, you can get too much of a good thing. I needed a better solution. I went searching out doctors again and at least the "hernia" was obvious and obviously split open again. Realizing that swift payment for the doctor was out of the question as was H-cap coverage I was in for another long wait. In fact I went directly to several local hospital administrators and all gave lip service and nothing else. In fact, one told me, off the record there was no way a hospital billing department would even consider the same H-cap operation on the same person in the same year as they were scared it would provoke an audit from the welfare department. It would be at least another 9 months before I would be H-cap eligible again.

Being desperate, I was able to seek out a kind person able to do a M*A*S*H style operation, on a back porch. The only anesthesia was a light shot of something smuggled out of a care facility and shot of whisky. Autistic's really don't feel all that much pain: as you now realize. The operation went incredibility smooth and the person doing the work was literally amazed. I was able to walk again, and if I wore the back braces I could do quite a bit. Almost a year to the day of the previous operation, I again had the hernia repaired and this time mesh was used, and all is "well." I often wondered if my pain tolerance has to do with being 'tough skinned'. It seems right below my skin surface is a layer of metal armor. Normal people seem to be made of skin and Jello thus their probably more attuned to bruises and feeing pain and cold and warm. I don't have a hard time feeling extreme hot or cold but luke warm for me is typically hot for others. Conversely, really cold, biting cold is almost oblivious to me. When out of doors in the winter the first stages of frostbite are really my first clue something is amiss.

After all of this unplanned medical experience I now wear Medical ID tags and suggest others do as well. Short of something real obvious or blood spurting, we are likely to be mistreated, considered not injured, or simply laughed at. My ID tags state **Autistic Disorder W/H associated pain tolerance. Needs a communication partner.** By now the pain tolerance is obvious enough but the communication is a necessity as well, even if the person can communicate effectively the Odd Medically Opposite story will throw many doctor nurses and EMT personal for a loop. Some one is needed to back-up the unbelievable. (I realize it might hard for an autistic person to wear the tags, but I got used to them, eventually)

As of this writing some 6 years after the injury, the repaired hernia is healed and now two more "oddly located muscle" tears need fixed. Technically there is nothing pinched in them so therefore they are not hernias but still I can stick my fingers in them. That instantly provokes a need to be sick. I can walk and stand for short periods of time but lifting is impossible as once down getting up with the added weight to contend with my legs simply can't lift all the weight. I end up just "shaking and shivering" and sometimes it will be half-an-hour before I can stand up with any ease.

Constant pain a really new experience for me is felt down the front of my legs and my heels and arches hurt almost all the time. Since the accident I have always had some hip pain but now it is constant, and again if an Autistic feels pain it must be bad. Most times 1/2 an aspirin can cure anything. If I'm really in pain my secret weapon is some high powered pain pills 1/2 pill and I don't feel a thing! I'm really thankful I do live at home since with out the security of being there and my family's fiscal help I'd be out on the street.

Sleepy Interns, Autism, & Useless Social Services

You would think in todays modern world lack of pain sensation wouldn't really be a major factor in health care, after all the there are Cat Scans, X-rays, and ultra-sounds among the many aids available to help point out trouble. Well providing you have insurance, at least. Granted many HMO's are very crude and rude and swamp their patient with all kind of unnecessary grief and in many cases sub-standard care but at least you have health care privileges. Thankfully, to you can probably claim your self-normal in terms of health care you feel pain you react correctly to exams and you are not labeled Autistic. As I alluded to in previous chapters normal emotional people, emotional thinkers, health care providers included, let their emotional minds tell them "oh no, what a piece of work, Autistic," "What's that, I don't know about that", "how is he going to pay?" etc. By the time the health care professional is in the exam room they have already decided not to deal effectively with my case, their goal often times is to refer me to another doctor or clinic, as quickly as possible. I had been discovering this for the last 5 years as well. I had published in my local paper the following essay that tells of the struggle.

Testing our social services

Rich Schull

Guest column

I generally cry when I read news that tells of America's fiscal aid to foreign countries. Whether helping to build power plants, covering bad debt or perhaps restore a castle in Ghana (Saturday, Dec. 14, in the *Eagle-Gazette's* Accent section). Often, "Yankee stay home" is how we are greeted.

Then I wonder about the $5.1 million expenditure in 1996 to build a third golf course at Andrews Air Force Base, along with the now famous toilet seats and the scores of other abuses.

Yet, the real America is one really in need of the expenditure. Our homeless and veterans are not the stereotypical drunk lazy bums. They are victims of the society in which they live. Social Security could use this money as well.

Five years ago after suffering serious injury, not only did I discover welfare to be useless but the social agencies as well. While the social services are staffed with caring people, their hands were tied to the policy and mostly Republican reform regulations currently in effect. Everybody off welfare, as the politicians say. That includes everyone — even those who need it.

I quickly found out after my injuries that, without insurance, medical care is impossible for close to a year. I limped along doing what the welfare department called a spend down. I had made just enough money in the previous year that I was not qualified for any version of welfare. Finally, after a years worth of unemployment, I was eligible for H-Cap (Hospital care assurance program) — a weak version of welfare. This is the only version of welfare available to a male older than 18, and it is income based.

To my dismay, I discovered H-Cap only covers the hospital charges, it does nothing in dealing with the doctor bills, anesthesiologists or pre-admission testing — all normal and customary procedures one needs before an operation. Try getting a doctor to

work for free. I was able to find a kind doctor who agreed to do the operation, providing I sold my last worthwhile possession (my Festiva) to pay his bill.

Thankfully I kept my old Mercury that still runs at 268,000 miles.

During this, my "discovery year," I realized that I was high functioning autistic. Actually I had been all my life and thankfully I had superior splinter skills which had enabled me to make a living to that point.

I had always been able to get by and I did make it through high school, taking many classes two or three times, but still I made it. College has left me short a degree despite taking chemistry four times. Autism is a birth defect that results in brain damage, as well as some physical limitations. Rain Man, the character portrayed by Dustin Hoffman in the movie of the same name is the stereotypical normal for autism. Being high functioning, I realize the scary difference. Being autistic and injured, as I discovered highlighted one of autism's most obvious points, that I don't feel physical pain.

For close to a year I suffered from and yet didn't feel the pain the normal person would have felt living with three hernias. I simply collapsed "in shock" and ended up in the emergency room usually for a pain shot and a kick out the door. Ironically, H-Cap covered the cost of my 12 ER visits in the past four years at a ridiculous cost to the taxpayers. The correct operation would have been cheaper, not to mention I'd be working again, paying taxes.

Not quite fully aware of my autism, I went back to work after the operation since I felt good and partly because the bill collectors from the other hospital services were relentless, rude and very consistent. I had a "need" to pay them off quickly. In reality I had gone back to work too soon

and again re-injured the fixed hernia.

I was back to hopeless again: I could hardly walk or stand. Again I was qualified for H-Cap and again it was worthless, as I had no means to pay for the other services. I was put into a clinic program offered by one of the hospital conglomerates in the area. In reality it was a nice way of saying no, get lost and have a nice day all at the same time.

It got to be a joke in our household when the phone call was going to come cancelling the appointment for whatever service it was they were going to offer.

Desperate for any relief I checked with other hospitals and caregivers and was given nothing but lip service. One administrator in a Columbus hospital told me if I could find a doctor to do the operation no hospital billing department would even consider doing the same operation on the same person in the same year, for provoking an audit from the welfare department. I was in for another year's wait.

Meanwhile, being desperate I was able to find a person able to do a M*A*S*H-style operation right here in Fairfield County. I'm glad it wasn't brain surgery. I was able to walk again. After the year wait, almost to the day I again had the same operation again and this time it was repaired with mesh and it has held. There are still two more hernias yet to be repaired.

Meanwhile, I considered my situation an applied for social security disability. Most other autistics receive SSDI. This also was a nightmare as the local MR/DD mental health system I was directed to by Social Security knew nothing of autism nor did a Columbus-based university. The university was especially pathetic in both their knowledge and manner. A psychologist, paid for by my dad, confirmed the autism.

I found out that I really do function very high and can count myself among the few autistics worldwide that can drive. The S.S. claim also brought about a physical that found nothing wrong. When two points of autism

were brought up, including the lack of pain sensation, I was simply laughed at.

Real-world testing, used to predict how I might be expected to survive on my own, showed that — all things considered — I didn't test well at all in some situations. In fact I had some terrible scores, as well as some very good ones. However I was still qualified to work in fast food one-half day per week, thus I'm ineligible for SSDI.

The Social Security SSDI determining process is a fine example of government in action all my testing, interviews, etc., all took less than a month in total time spent directly dealing with the claim. It was often several months before the next step in the process was scheduled, and nothing got done between Thanksgiving and New Year's Day. Worse yet, if the approval you needed to progress on to the next stage in the process and the paperwork needed for it was sitting on someone's desk that had a month's vacation, well guess what, you waited. My total claim time was 1.5 years.

I have found a new clinic program that promises the operation I need. It will be done by interns. There I have found a wonderful doctor that is taking the time to learn about autism. In an effort to find the trouble, he has scheduled a "cat scan" in hopes it will help pinpoint the trouble. As of this writing, I'm still several days from the scan, still plenty of time for them to cancel.

I applaud the recent *Eagle-Gazette* articles about poverty and those of us living on the edge. If I didn't live at home, I'd be on the street without hope. I'm sure most readers of this would agree welfare reform has gone too far and, in reality, does nothing to help those who really need it.

Even worse when I qualify for my $5- to $6-an-hour job, if it offers insurance, the odds are I won't qualify as those with autism are not covered.

So much for a kinder gentler nation.

(Rich Schull is a resident of Carroll.)

3-1-99 - CAT SCAN FILMS WERE FINALLY READ BY SELF AND the SHATTERED HIP JOINT AND DEFORMED RIB CAGE WERE OBVIOUS. OTHER DOCTORS HAVE CONFIRMED THIS .T CARMEL CLINIC REFUSED to RE READ the X-RAYS, AND I HAD to OBTAIN the FILMS UNDER FALSE PRETENSE.

71

Testing our Social Services   Guest column Lancaster   Eagle-Gazette 1-8-99

All politics aside, the system really doesn't work any matter who tries to fiddle with it. The person in my situation and those like it are put into the "de-fault mode", meaning to health care providers, get rid of them, hide them or "deal" with them. The clinic program I deal with is trying so hard to do nothing afraid to spend a buck. If all that effort was channeled in a different direction, "boy" the difference it might make. These folks are pro at canceling appointments right as your leaving the house and then re-scheduling them 3–4 months later. If their computers could go 6 months the appointment would be scheduled then. I missed my appointment cancellation once arrived at the hospital and was told the doctor was "out of town", 'out of town' must mean the hospital cafeteria as I had just seen the doctor in question entering it a I was entering the hospital for my appointment.

Once you do see a doctor they really don't look too hard to find anything wrong but that is hardly a surprise as the visit is "free", actually H-cap pays for it. The doctors have typically been ignorant of Autism (not a surprise) and not willing to take the time to understand it. Or they have been so sleepy they were hardly walking and if were not for the pills they prescribed themselves they'd been out cold. Passing the patient is a popular pastime for these intern run clinics, if something is too hard to deal with send it to another clinic or doctor. Occasionally, I do get a good doctor at heart that really takes an interest in Autism and the odd medicine it entails but sadly that intern typically makes waves in the system as I see it and is suddenly "no longer my doctor"

That indeed was the case with the CAT Scan. It actually took me 5 years to get it and according to the clinic nothing was abnormal in it, that may be, but the sleepy doctors in charge of reading it are probably not ineffable, and worse yet the clinic is the one in charge of telling you "nothings wrong" are the ones that would be responsible for the care and giving it out. There reputation precedes them; actions really do speak louder than words. When I asked for a second reading of the Cat Scan it fell on death ears, and suddenly my "Special" intern that was doing better than average is no longer available to me. Hells fire, he was probably fired for doing something correctly. On false pretenses I obtained copies of the films and was APPALED when I seen the obvious shattered hip joint and deformed Rib Cage just looking at them with a desk lamp. My Doctor confirmed my readings.

I'm sure if I'd had access to normal care and insurance all would be fixed and healed by now. Granted the HMO would have been screaming you can't have a Cat Scan for a hernia as it wouldn't be normal and customary and it would take a million approvals from all kind of doctors and maybe even your dog. But, all I really needed was few X-rays and treatment (I suspect) something that is entirely beyond the clinical medical science.

As you can see the best of today's care is often not available. Then when the Autistic person doesn't react properly to the exam or shows no pain, the assumption is nothing wrong. Just how many patients after all don't react to pain? Then typically a really strange injury is unbelievable, and Autistic explanations I dare say hardly ever communicate the point of a conversation, especially a fast paced one in a doctor's office. Additionally, I have found by talking to other Autistics they usually have little idea that their pain threshold is so much greater than the normal, thus they no idea of what pain really is OR how to react to it. It is such a concept to them that its discovery will have to be left to first hand discovery of it. I sincerely hope others don't have to find out what it is about, but if you do please keep this writing in mind, and again wear medical ID tags.

Just imagine the benefits to society if the reason for our pain tolerance could be figured out and some drug or treatment is created to duplicate it. Those in pain especially constant pain might be able to re-gain control of their lives, without having to be addicted to something. I especially hope the people at the opposite end of the pain spectrum those suffering from Cluster Headaches who have to take presciption morphine for a headache could be the first to benefit. I list the Cluster Headache web site in the reference section of this book.

Sadly, that last idea is nothing more than a Pandora's box. I firmly believe the medical community could in no way be trusted to carefully and respectfully carry out experiments on Autistic patients in the name of research. There is just too much chance of abuse and people ending up like the character of the movie Elephant man. A few permanently hurt Autistic people would be a small price to pay for the millions in profit available from a cure from pain. The typical Autistic would be at a horrible dis-advanatage not being able to communicate effectively.

I even invited Washington to get on the act,

DAVID L. HOBSON
7TH DISTRICT, OHIO

WASHINGTON OFFICE
1514 Longworth HOB
Washington, DC 20515

(202) 225-4324

CONGRESS OF THE UNITED STATES
HOUSE OF REPRESENTATIVES

COMMITTEE ON APPROPRIATIONS

SUBCOMMITTEES:
MILITARY CONSTRUCTION
CHAIRMAN
DEFENSE
VA, HUD, AND INDEPENDENT AGENCIES

ASSISTANT MAJORITY WHIP

March 4, 1999

Rich Schull
5960 High St NW
Carroll, OH 43112-9771

Dear Rich:

Thank you for writing and sending a copy of your article published in the Lancaster Eagle-Gazette. It was good to know your thoughts on welfare reform, social security, and health care, and I am sorry about your difficult experience in obtaining health care.

I agree that many Americans need to receive better health care coverage. The pendulum in health care has moved too far toward controlling costs and has placed too much control in the hands of the insurance companies. This shift toward controlling costs has often been at the expense of patient care. For that reason, I actively participated in and helped write the Health Insurance Portability and Accountability Act (HIPAA) of 1996 (P.L. 104-191). HIPAA is the first step in increasing the availability and renewability of health insurance coverage for certain employees and individuals. It also limits the use of preexisting condition restrictions.

Even though the application of HIPAA has not lived up to expectations, the market approach is still the best answer to health care. Accordingly, I was pleased when former Speaker Newt Gingrich (R-GA) asked me to participate in a Congressional Leadership Health Care Group to come up with a balanced approach to improve health care services and protect patients. On July 16, 1998, the Leadership Working Group introduced the *Patient Protection Act* (H.R. 4250). H.R. 4250 allows health care consumers to choose their own health care professional, appeal denied claims to an impartial third party, receive emergency care coverage when it is generally believed to be necessary, and hold health plans accountable for their work.

H.R. 4205 was passed by the House of Representatives by a vote of 216 Yeas to 210 Nays on July 24, 1998. Unfortunately, the Senate did not pass HMO reform legislation in the 105th session of Congress. Nevertheless, both the Speaker of the House of Representatives, Dennis Hastert (R-IL), and the Majority Leader, Dick Armey (R-TX), have made health care reform a priority in the current session (the 106th) of Congress. Rest assured that I will actively participate in this debate and will remember your situation.

Again, thanks for writing. Please do not hesitate to let me know whenever I can help.

Sincerely,

DAVID L. HOBSON
Member of Congress

Thanks for sending
the article.

SPRINGFIELD OFFICE
5 W. North St., Sta. 200
P.O. Box 269
Springfield, OH 46501-0269

(937) 325-0474

THIS STATIONERY PRINTED ON PAPER MADE OF RECYCLED FIBERS

LANCASTER OFFICE
212 S. Broad St.
Room 55
Lancaster, OH 43130-4389

(740) 654-5149

10

Finding a Doctor

Finding a medical doctor is a pretty big task! It most likely is impossible at this point, Autism is hardly known about and it is strange and opposite of normal medicine reality makes the average doctor cringe. Then again, the Autistic "is hardly hurt" most live such a sheltered life that major injury is a lot less likely to happen. In my case the common injuries I have experienced as an auto mechanic and in normal life have a story to tell all of their own. Many have proved to be beyond medical treatment either out of ignorance on the part of the Autistic and doctor or both, surly an insurance company someplace has done their part in preventing Autistic health care, as well.

My 1st experience with doctors that claimed to have some expertise with Autism left me feeling cheated. I heard several of the parties in question speak at an Autism gathering and couldn't help but want to scream. I got the impression from one of the speakers that she/he was out to be first to discover something, thus the get their names in the history books. Autism has enough heroes'—I have little respect for someone exploiting the people and the cause. Another experience a personal one was particularly fowl. The party in question had somewhat of a local reputation for be an respected expert in Autism and the truth be told she/he was the only one in the area that even dealt with Autistic persons and I'm sure (I HOPE) I was the only adult s/he ever seen. I really feel for his typical patient most likely a child that has little or no effect regarding his/her health care. Questionable practices and poor preference even if realized by an Autistic child and related to his parent or caregiver would most likely be discounted at the least and shrugged off as dislike for doctors in general thus this questionable quack in my opinion floats along getting rave reviews. Even the worst performance with out a critic becomes legendary. As you know from reading this far in the book Autistics don't feel pain correctly, so this doctor, a psychologist decides to practice physical medicine and probes my sides trying to find the hernia's. Of Course, I showed no reaction instantly and after we set down I had the feeling of having to throw up: I

came to my senses and quit trusting this doctor thus I thought, If s/he was ignorant of the point Autistic's didn't feel pain, what else didn't s/he know? In fact s/
he was bemoaning the fact s/he couldn't find the hernias and I was faking not
only the hernias but also the entire Autism experience.

Yet other experiences lead to me to think, some of the worst doctors in medicine
or maybe the boldest choose a speciality where their not likely to be critiqued or
questioned and if they are, circumstances surrounding the event lean in their
favor. Autism the research of or the practice of certainly offers the Swiss Bank
account type of practice for the unscrupulous brand of doctor. Of course, I'm
sure there are fine doctors about that deal with Autistics and to those good guys
please don't take offense to my comments but rather help us rid ourselves of the
questionable doctors within the spectrum.

I've searched high and low to find an Autism doctor using the resources of the
Autism Society of America and the Via the Internet, I found the listings of the
Autism Research Institute, there; I did find a large list of doctors that would see
Autistic Patients. I found two here in Ohio and several others within driving distance. (Sadly I couldn't afford the visits) The Autism Society had fewer listings in
general and could offer me nothing. I had heard years ago that the ASA and the
Autism Research Institute seemed to be on different playing fields but, it never
really sunk in, just how far apart they are, until this. I found the needed information in literality minutes on the ARI website. What I can't figure is if both organizations fly the same banner of "Lets help the Autistic", why is it the common
everyday basic knowledge such as doctors list can't at least be shared among the
non-profit organizations. At the least provide a link to each other's websites and
publications. Granted from what I seen the two organizations are coming from
two different points of view but still that is no reason to risk the care of someone
autistic just because, dare I say two different EMOTIONAL parties can't work
with one another. This is a prime example of emotional thinking, Gee, I hope I
didn't damage any ego's here. Some of these same groups and others also ignored
all my efforts in contacting them for help with this book.

On a related note I did discover many ways I could leave my body to Autism
research (or medical research) while doing the doctor search. It seems they want
to do a lot for you when you're dead but what, about the living? Although I have
not totally ruled the idea out and after all I should help the cause of Autism as
much as possible. But I have experienced so much bad medicine and double standards it doesn't seem worth it. I even give-up my organ donor card some time ago

as a result of the poor medicine and appalling lack of concern I experienced during this Autistic ordeal. Here of late the clinic I dealt with now advertises all over the city "You Would be Amazed at What We Do?" no I wouldn't I've had the M*A*S*H operation and set in your clinics been "treated" by your doctors and experienced your appointment policy.

The double standard of care is never more obvious than the clinic I dealt with: It is run by the same hospital conglomerate that the rest of my insured family uses. After their operations they get follow-up phone calls asking if one is allright? How the service was? Etc. I answered one of those calls just last month and pretended to be dad. They were calling about a heart operation that had just been completed on him and instead I answered on my behalf. The shocked person (Maybe a Volunteer) on the other end of the line was in disbelief, as I never gave a higher rating than a 5 on a 10 scale. When she figured out I was referring to my 14 canceled (by the hospital) clinic appointments I heard her rip up the form she was filling out. I'm glad I don't have cancer they would tell me it doesn't spread.

Visiting the Doctor......Warnings, Suggestions and Hope.

If one has been lucky enough to find a doctor, the rather extreme ideals we have been discussing such as shock as the only symptom, or simply not being able to move are often the first sign something is amiss. In reality the dis-located hip has been causing trouble for months (moods for example) and yet the patient was still walking on it. Pain for an Autistic is merely confusion; after all it has hardly ever been felt and its use as a diagnostic tool is limited in our case. Of course this totally confuses the caregiver and the parent who have all adjusted to the fact the more it hurts the worse it hurts the more serious the injury or illness. The normal person has the luxury of nature's early warning system and pain pinpointing that can lead to the correct treatment and even operations. The autistic is either "all go" or fully stopped there is little in between and if someone autistic feels constant pain there is something really wrong. I haven't taken 30 aspirin in my life, and even after surgery I only needed three pain pills.

When I study my early days as an auto mechanic, I frequently recall breaking nuts and bolts due to overt-tightening. It became necessary for me to always use a torque wrench, and I began to train myself to 'feel' the appropriate amount of tightening. Checking the previous work I didn't break, I discovered it was consistently over torqued by 20 to 30 FT. Lbs. This lack of sensory perception may be related to my in-ability to feel pain. I suspect my tactile sensory perception may only be 60%, compared to that of the average person. When I shave with a straight razor I have to *feel* by looking in the mirror to get an idea of just how hard I'm pressing. If I'm not real careful I really cut my self-deep. It feels to me like I'm not putting any pressure at all on the razor and it shouldn't be working. Besides the noise I prefer electric razors they seem more suited to the situation.

Doctors and nurses will face some of the strangest circumstances and patients of their careers when dealing with the autistic. All normal medicine and procedures seem useless since the pain that offers a clue isn't there to or not powerful enough to induce a reaction. Additionally, the Autistic patient doesn't communicate well and often what he trying to say or point out is mis-understood. Doctors and nurses should make an effort to speak softly and slowly and try not to use big words when talking to the patient. The word "dehabilitationing" for example might be very confusing to an Autistic patient. It is due to the fact a word like that requires a lot of processing, not that they don't understand it, eventually they will figure it out, usually after the visit is over.

Autistics please realize your medically opposite of normal, and try to the help the doctor and nurse by answering their questions and please let them do most of the talking, there trying to pinpoint the trouble. Don't be surprised if the diagnosis or treatment seem different than what you expected. Remember they are "flying blind." Even if the treatment is incorrect it won't be a wasted experience, as it will have ruled out another possibility. Also remember the limited pain you experience with an injury usually disappears as fast as, it presented itself. Therefore it is vital for the autistic to remember where the pain was felt. In our case do indeed "lie "and fake pain during the exam, even if we act a little "too good" it just might make the difference between treatment or being sent off. Do this especially if the doctor is not known to you and you're sure he is unaware of Autism. In fact nowadays should I have to see a doctor I don't even tell them of the Autism it just scares them, and I put on a "good show". I have a good enough idea of the pain that if I act it out: I'm more likely to be treated correctly.

The Polaroid Photo Syndrome

The following analysis refers to and compares to the Polaroid Land cameras that self develop their own pictures to an Autistic getting an injury. I'm sure all of you have seen the photo develop a time or two. In this case we will consider a slightly out of focus completed picture. A parallel concept to the Polaroid, is the Autistic that just might have been injured.

"SNAP" the red button is pushed all kinds of things happen and the picture comes out all blank. *"SNAP" the autistic has just caught a heavy falling object, all kinds of things happen. The Autistic is lying on the ground experiencing all kind of different feeling, maybe even pain.*

The Picture starts to turn from grey nothing to images. *The Autistic realizes he can't get up and parts of his body are immobile. Slowly, the pain subsides and he starts to move and stretch, eventually he stands up.* (911 would have been called for anyone else)

The photo is now looking like something; the colors are becoming apparent, as are the shapes and the background. *At this point the autistic only if badly hurt realizes that he might need stitches, or have broken bones, or If he is really "lucky" blood might be spurting giving a clue to where he is hurt. In reality he probably has done some major injury and has no idea t is wrong, or even if there is anything askew.*

The photo is finally developed and it came out blurry, the object of the shot is recognizable to those who know what it is but the ignorant person seeing the shot for the first time might not figure it out. *The autistic by now knows something is wrong, since doing anything major results in symptoms of shock. A general idea of the injury is enjoyed, but the specifics of how bad the pain is, where it is centered are all beyond his grasp. Just like the developed out of focus photo.*

Doctor's and Autistic in your office is doable but obviously, the results or the means of achieving them might be different. First off contrary to what you have been taught, when doing an exam pushing harder and harder in a suspected area usually has no results. Initially at least. Often after an exam more is felt (delayed reaction) and although the pain would probably not be severe it is very irritating and more noticeable. It might be a good idea to keep the patient in the office after the exam as something might develop in a half-hour or so. A better Exam might be a light pressure rub over the area. Lightly rub your hand over the area and let the patient translate what is felt, remember our sensitive skin? Let it do what it will in this case.

Remember an Autistic lives in his body all the time and is attuned to it more than anyone can be, he is aware of the different from normal feelings and probably realizes to some extent where they are coming from. It might help if the patient is given magic markers and told to draw what he feels or has felt directly on his body. For example, Red markers could pinpoint where s/he might be feeling constant pain a different color could be used to point out a specific wound lump etc. Once in "war paint" the injuries might be more apparent. A *reverse exam*, where the patient points out on the doctor himself where it hurts is really helpful to it will allow the doctor to translate for himself some of what the patient is feeling. I did this reverse exam at the suggestion of my M*A*S*H surgeon by rubbing my hands over the same spot on the surgeon using my fingertips to locate the severe pain and hand pressure to simulate the pain of the general area. The surgeon was amazed the outcomes and had no idea just how severe the pain was. Another thing you might do is recreate the injury, in your mind possibly, if one fell out of a tree think how the normal child might be reacting? Give the Autistic plenty of time to think of the correct answer to your questions, I find our slow thought process results in de-fault answers that are not always correct. Another favor? Please get rid of the paper on the exam table. It is loud and painful to Autistic hearing, and affects the thought process.

Some updates

Before this goes to press some years after the injuries none of them have been repaired most of them have kind of healed on their own. The hip still turns black and blue, after doing too much. This might shock my readers but the right" hernia" that NO doctor could find or would admit to now spurts blood right out through the skin when I do to much. In a way that is good I can deal with the blood leaking as since the bleeding stated I feel lots better. Of course there is no reason to go the doctor when all he could do is recommend tests and other doctors all are beyond my budget. Of course H-Cap if I qualified would only pay for the Hospital and nothing else. I dare you to get doctors appointment with out a bank account or insurance.

The latest medical disaster ended on a good note but it is every bit as scary as the others. The X-ray below was the talk of the ER as all were amazed to see the needle in my foot. The lady that developed and first looked at the film was shell shocked and said with a little stagger in her voice "You have a needle in your foot". Indeed I had and that wasn't the worst of it. The needle had been in my foot since the previous day and I had walked on it all day at work and didn't feel it nor did I feel it go in my foot. I did feel my foot get stuck on the carpet and simply pulled the needle from my foot, and when about my business. The needle as it turns out was bigger than average and ¼ of it had broken off in my foot. When I awoke the next morning I seen the foot was swelled and it was finally getting sore.

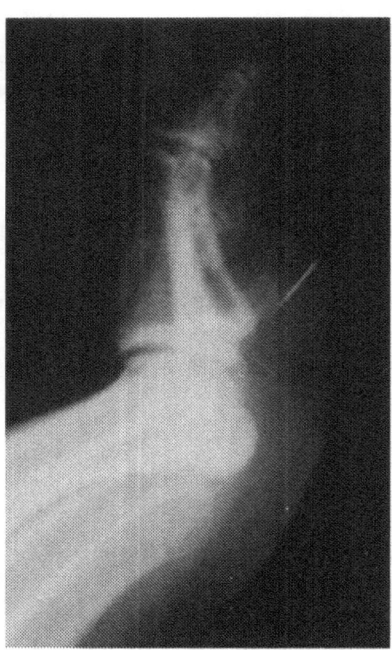

The needle is obvious and again I didn't feel it! Only after I walked on it for a day and infection was setting in did I feel anything at all. The only reason I knew it went in was it stopped my foot in its tracks and I thought I pulled all of it out, but it was a bigger needle than normal.

This is proof positive we need X-rays as the first line of diagnosis. I have heard from others the world over with broken elbows, fractured wrist and ankles all treated as sprains or more minor injuries! If It didn't hurt how could it be broken?

IF we feel anything at all it is twice a severe as it would be in a normal person, the tummy ache we do feel would have you laying flat in the hospital.

The ER as I mentioned was filled with X-ray lookers and by this time I knew enough to tell them I was Autistic and didn't feel pain. With the X-ray clearly proving the needle was in the foot I was given a Tetanus shot, the wound was cleaned and I was told to get lost and call a surgeon on Monday. Well, as usual a budget with out money keeps the doors of medicine shut and I didn't want to go through the clinic experience again and figured it would be easier to remove the needle my self now that I seen the X-ray. This simple operation I did myself naturally went well and I even gave my self-a stitch as the wound ended up being bigger than I expected.

Mental Health

There is a statement for you, Frankly I'm amazed I have any sanity left at all. After all, I have dealt with a few too many Autism experts many of whom are "trained professionals", but still I wonder? Granted the worst offenders in my case were working for "free" usually under the terms of welfare or social security which in a similar vain to the clinic health care I spoke of earlier and of the same low caliber.

One really pathetic example of free psychological health care was from a state university here in central Ohio. I was sent to this institution, during the Social Security disability determining process. Actually I contacted them myself before the Social Security did and thus had the process of the evaluation already started by the time the official paperwork caught up. Never the less this is where I'd been sent by Social Security. That action alone saved several months in the one-and-a-half year claim process.

The two-day evaluation on separate Fridays was done by a somewhat locally known autism "expert." Actually this person was probably the only "expert" in Autism in central Ohio, and it seemed as if the title and status of the person in question was earned by default. The doctor was more worried that I learned of Autism via the radio program, on "that liberal NPR" and thus I was trying to get on to welfare on the delusion that I was Autistic. Additionally, the religious beliefs of the doctor were painfully evident as the doctor said some key words with a smear in the voice. During the interviews the doctor turned around everything I said used it against me belittling all of my accomplishments we talked of. Even if this was "approved" psychological practice it was certainly bad manners. Normal thinkers don't know it but what they say and how they say it are two different things. I bet autistic hears the slight imperfections in their voices that usually later prove to be true indicators of what was really being thought.

As it happened dad was requested to go along on the final interview and he to realized the joker mentality of this "doctor." After our letter of complaint was sent registered mail to the place in question it must have hit home as I seen by accident a few months later a 'special report' in my files during the physical exam (for ssdi) when a folder was left open by accident. The report was from the 'medical review and procedures' board, and proclaimed that the psychologists physical was proper just and performed correctly. My research into that board later determined that it is an advisory committee of other doctors that review such cases: that is a bit like asking your dog if you did something bad?

As expected the results were my Autism was delusional, and my life would be perfect if I *went to church*. And quit being gay. If the doctor would have had the insight to read the psychological report about me sent from an intensive evaluation done by my local MR/DD center he would have never made such flippant remarks. When I offered my 60-page autobiography in an effort to help in the evaluation I was told it wasn't necessary. The final summery given by the doctor actually did start out "we like to get paid for our work", funny I thought tax dollars funded this institution.

On a brighter note my local MR/DD mental health board really did a fine job in helping, but frankly they were too overworked dealing with child abuse, domestic violence and drinking to figure out Autism, and they bravely admitted they knew little of Autism and I should go elsewhere. They were also delighted that I had handled the oeriention question so effectively. They did agree something was wrong but had no real clue to what was up. A private psychologist paid for by my dad in another state confirmed the Autism. It was worth the 3-or 4, 6 hour trips, and one way for the visits. It was a pleasure too not to have to explain Autism to the professional you were seeing. The picture explanations were unnecessary, as was the explanation of the lack of pain sensation and the over feeling of the skin. These key points were the main topics of conversation at the other places I'd been, it was all news to them.

This psychologist read my autobiography listened intently and never made rude comments and if we disagreed it was handled in a suitable manor. The final out come was PDD/NOS atypical autism. I was 35 at the time.

Susan J. Rautio-Dietz, Ph.D.   *Psychologist*

The Morgan House   Health Service Provider
532 N. Walnut St., Suite D
P.O. Box 5185
Bloomington, Indiana 47407-5185

DSM-IV

Asperger's Disorder   #299.80

(aka Atypical Autism or
PDD NOS [Pervasive Developmental
Disorder Not Otherwise Specified])

(with somaticization and avoidant
personality)

The official diagnosis

One more evaluation sponsored by the Judge in charge of hearing my social security claim was to determine just how I would survive in the real world. The real world testing was done in a Small southern Ohio town and consisted of a mini psychological interview and the Iowa Basic test that I taken ever since grade school and even mentioned in one of the questions the Panama Canal in the context that we still had control over it. Further another question was, the *bible* is a good book to read? I'm sure I got that one wrong as I answered all 5 blanks at once as protest. At the very least it is a politically charged question, and has no business in an IQ test. (I believe the copyright was 1969) I guess the tests were still valid if not a little out of date.

The result form this real world testing showed I did good in some things and horrible in others and they really did mirror real life to a great degree. As usual I had terrible math skills and social reasoning. In the end I was qualified from the results of this test to work in fast food ½ day per week even with injuries and that seems to be the "standard" to meet if you get Social Security disability these days. I was told, off the record, "at one time not all that long ago I'd been approved" by a social security worker. I never really had intentions of a life of social security. But, rather I was trying for it for the insurance it would have offered. Despite Autism I can do some pretty major work in the right environment, but I have to be able to walk first.

Yet another layer in this nightmare is the Department Of Rehabilitation Services, a state agency charged with helping re-train workers. Initially I was impressed with them (after I waited for 6 months to be moved to the top of the queue.) I was quickly approved for their job training and other services which included the purchase of the 'hearing aid filters' I spoke of earlier. Eventually one appointment lead to another and soon they are cancelling appointments and sometimes they didn't even tell me. I finally quit pressuring them. Then suddenly I got a call from them, stating that I hadn't been seen in a awhile and we need to get something going. They had this seemingly imagnary dead line to meet where all kinds of paperwork needed to be turned in again; we complied. This dead line was suspiciously close to the end of a fiscal year. It was full 4 months before I heard from them again and this time they suspended their services until my medical problems were taken of. Of course were still working on that one.

As I'm sure you can relate, the social services are seriously deficient in a number of respects. The red tape bureaucracy and the 'cut funding' along with the in general poor attitude of the overworked providers all result in basically nothing. I suspect in this day and age no 'High Functioning Person' would qualify for a thing and one would be better off making your own plan. My 1.5 year Struggle with the SSDI claim was wasted time and if were not for the fact we had a SSDI lawyer on the case we might still be perusing the case up the wrong tree. In the end we were urged to drop the case as the Social Security judge overseeing my case was rumored to be so strict and crude that she would kick her own mother out onto the street. A second atty. confirmed this. Had we had a different judge it still might have been worth the effort.

11

Autistic Driving

I thought long and hard on the content of this book and decided I would be doing a great injustice to the experiment if I failed to include my driving experience I wondered to my self on this and many other subjects if they should be brought up at all but and decided to include things purely in terms of the experiment and the results of it. Readers to this point of the book that are just getting acquainted for the first time with Autistic thought are probably confused and maybe horrified that someone Autistic even entertain the thought of driving. Maybe some of these people are of the mentality that group homes are the only place for someone Autistic.

Driving as your aware is one of the easier tasks in life and many normal drivers often forget the responsibility of driving safely. How many people do you see talking on the phone etc.? Driving can be a simple predictable task in 98% of all cases, paying total attention to your driving like someone Autistic has to do would result in a more accident free world. I even go so far in driving as to plan my trips to avoid left turns, if possible and avoid notably dangerous intersections.

Deciding on weather or not to allow an Autistic person to drive is a important personal decision, and each case would have to decided on a case by case basis. Generally I feel a high-functioning person might make a good driver providing the differences between a normal and an Autistic driver are realized and respected. I know of many Autistic drivers diagnosed high-functioning. Additionally via my Internet web site I have met a number of people, usually parents and close relatives of someone Autistic that probably would have been diagnosed in school providing Autism was diagnosable in earlier times, which drive as well. I always tease my friend Tony in Australia that if he learned to drive on the "wrong" side of the road, "anyone could do that!" Of course, the comment is returned. It Is the Right turns "downunder" that will get you vs. America's Left turns.

My first advice to an Autistic person who wishes to drive is to have his or her eyes checked for color blindness. As a beginner driver I was involved in many more accidents than the average beginner. Consistently, I seemed to having trouble with red and brown cars or objects. Although I did have the ability to see these colors, it was below the average person's ability. I also find that Red Brown color blindness is fairly common among the driving population as well. Whenever I drove my Red Truck or Luella I always have a disproportionate number of close calls when other drivers can't seem coming as easily. The non-autistic driver would probably not have been bothered by my slight problem with reds and browns. For an autistic driver however, where the processing is a few milliseconds slower, even a small disability can be serious. I've now trained myself to look for these colors, and reds and browns no longer give me grief. I also cheat now and wear yellow or green lenses (sunglasses) while driving. This changes the color of the world to yellow and thus highlights reds. Some Autistics also suffer from Irlen's syndrome another vision disorder, Web Sites can be found explaining that.

Another distracting factor while driving was the car radio. I found I became a safer driver, more alert driver by leaving the car radio turned off. Remember that these discoveries were made long before I was diagnosed autistic. Another "trick" I mentioned in the discussion on noise was a super quiet car. I added insulation, rubber (rust proofing) sound deadening to the door panels roof and floor as well as 'house" insulation and foam rubber to about every place in the car. I wonder if my really quiet Ford Festivia might have bounced if it were ever in an accident with the aid of all that extra cushioning. The quiet really made driving a pleasure and I no longer 'jumped' in a startled state when rock hit the bottom of the car, in fact I hear very few of them at all, any more. Before this when driving this car I'd be tooling along and an occasional stone would fly up and 'PING' under the car someplace as it was good for a tense moment or two. Note, if I were driving on a gravel road it didn't bother me at all to hear all the stones hitting under the car as I was driving on a gravel road after all, it was the smooth black top road with the occasional stone that done the deed.

Fortunately for me growing up in the country gave me plenty of learning opportunities. The Relative safety and slower speed of tractors, riding mowers and go-carts helped familiarize me with motorized vehicles Even riding a bicycle helped adjust me to movement and motion. Also, lightly traveled country roads made an easier transition for me when I began driving cars. The heavy traffic of any large urban area can be daunting even for the non-autistic driver, but it is doable.

Today I live in town and it has made me realize that I really long for the country and its easier driving. Between the passing Boom Boxes and loud cars in general and the city driving experience is much more work than pleasure. Every Autistic driver should start in the country and work their way up to driving in the city.

While driving I live by the "2 second" rule. If my vision detours to a mental thought picture, I force my self to return to optical vision, again I feel only 30% of my thoughts are normal with out pictures. The pictures these days only appear when I need to think about something, normal vision and reaction are common 98% of the time while driving. Autistic driving need not be difficult, providing the distractions are kept to a minimum. That means no radio of course or talking passengers and in fact, I ask my passengers to ride quietly except when giving directions and warnings. I also make an effort to avoid looking at the shinny spinning truck wheels as I go by them, I guess we really never totally get over spinning things. Night driving is helps as there is less information to process making other drivers are more obvious to me against a dark featureless background, and thus I am better able to anticipate their moves.

When traveling to new destinations, I will often memorize the names of the streets and the general layout of the area, names of the communities on the map before starting out. This way when I see the sign "Grove City" Dublin Etc. on a freeway sign I know what direction to go. I focus on street numbers a lot more than directions like 'turn right at the big tree'. Street numbers are at least ordered if not always easy to find. I also memorize the names of the streets I will be crossing and which one to turn on, and which one was 'too' far in the event I miss the turn. I also try to pay attention to the one way streets if they show on the map. I will use big landmarks, as guides occasionally providing it something really obvious like a filling station. My mental maps: picture thought complete with "computer animation" are pretty good at keeping me from getting lost.

With my driving self-analysis and the use of the Autistic driving standards, I feel quite comfortable driving. Autistics who must work harder to focus, may very well be better drivers than non-autistic that take far more liberties than they should while driving. Travel any freeway during rush hour, and it is not unusual to see drivers sipping coffee, chatting on the phone, applying make-up, reading a map, yelling at the kids, singing along to the radio, or attempting to prevent their dog from jumping from seat to seat. The Autistic knows better.

Defensive Driving

Since I discovered my color blindness, I have not had an accident. Thanks to my pictures I was able to avoid one. Understanding of normal thought and thinking 'told' me this person's actions and what they were likely to be, so I was able to figure out what I need to do to avoid the other drivers normal actions/and miss the accident. Actually, lots of things a normal person does really fit a pattern and a mold whether it is driving a car or doing a conversation. Only someone Autistic would have this prospective on normal people as spent our lives not only figuring out autism but normal thought as well. Anyway, a driver whose attention was distracted by an accident ran a light and I was directly in her path. I let my pictures develop, with the point of view being above the traffic looking down. (*This seemed to be an automatic process as was the View from above*) my mind was calculating the angle of the approaching car to mine, where the impact would occur and the potential severity of the impact. I found the results unsatisfactory.

Every time the wheels locked up in my (*thought*) picture, as would happen if I slammed on the brakes, the results became worse as the cars continued forward. The wheels continuing to spin offered the greatest control. (*I had a thought picture of a race car accident that I seen on TV some years back where the driver that missed the accident never applied the brakes*) Thus contrary to hitting the brakes, throwing up my arms and screaming, as most **emotional** thinkers would have done, I pressed hard on the gas pedal. Again, as mentioned earlier PANIC doesn't seem to be an automatic function for someone Autistic. After the event I have a little bit of "withdraw" if you will but, nothing during it.

The most control I could have over the impending accident was to attempt to locate the car differently than would have been possible by using the brakes. I calculated that even if I was hit the resulting collision would be minor, as the point of impact (*in my picture thoughts*) would have been different from head on and more in likely taken shape in my rear fender and the other drivers front one, All better alternatives than head on. The accident was narrowly avoided probably by millimeters. There was enough on demand power to move me out of harms way. The only causality to this was that the differential on my car started thumping after the near miss. With then 230,000 miles of wear I was not surprised. I did not complain.

GO figure, all of that insight and correctly paced fast thought literally saved an accident but yet the simplest of social situations, jobs and simple communication

fail me quite a bit of the time. Of course those thoughts didn't have to be translated to "English", analyzed for content, or explained to anyone. I was simply
thinking naturally with picture thought. See it does work! Just as you can't think
in pictures easily I'd have a hard time thinking normally. That is why you flour-
ish in most social situations you are doing and thinking in your natural language.

For some Autistics I could see everyday driving, to work for example might be
more doable, than say a trip to a new destination. The same destination everyday
and the same route traveled could be followed almost daily. However, I would
make it point to experience alternate routes, some time the original route will be
closed. Otherwise, I find it important to equip the car with cruise control, that
makes driving easier, as the speed is automatic and that helps to limit the looks
necessary to check the speed. Again the less distraction the better.

I love driving my old Pontiac and even earn a living driving rental cars to and
from various airport locations. Amazingly I even drive sometimes with loud passengers riding with me, but since it is the same route time and again it seems to
be more of a routine than driving. Still I always drive carefully and think more
than normal driver might about the trip and respect the responsibility of driving
effectively. My 30% functioning normal mind is working near capacity doing
this job and it is not at all boring for me. I suspect the average thinker would be
dizzy and board stiff doing a job like this. On the other hand my 70% Autistic
mind is board stiff and I have to work awfully hard to keep all kind of picture
thought from developing. All I need to hear is a vacuum leak or a noise and
instantly my picture thoughts are (want to be) busy picturing things like the engineering drawings of the leaking heater control switch, the running motor with a
faulty timing belt or the electrical fault in the cruise control.

I firmly believe Autistics that know the ins and outs of their Picture Thoughts
will make good drivers. If normal thought can be developed to a useable point I
can see most everyone being able to drive. We would always have to respect our
built in differences and really treat driving as an extreme privilege, kind of like
driving a Rolls Royce.

12

A Bit More Enlightenment

There are many important messages in this book ranging from the vital picture thought to pain tolerance and the many dealing with our state of mind and being. In my case it was my natural comfortable oerineration and coming to terms with that issue that made my Autistic success possible. To those who think I have taken terrible liberties by mixing gay and Autism too often through out this book, It was just part of the process and a necessary element of this blind backward Autism experiment. Just as you can NOT turn 'straight' off is part of you. It is your culture. Gay, Lesbian, Transgendered and Bisexual is part of us our culture and also cannot be turned off or hidden thus that is why it was inter-mixed with the Autism. You must admit it brought to light all kinds of ideas never thought of before. Perhaps you might be a pretty narrow-minded psycholo-gist, Autism researcher, Doctor or someone high up in autism circles. It might be hard to admit that you had a 'no brainier' sexual development experience grow-ing up. The world revolves about the straight lifestyle so you never had any learn-ing experience coping with something different. Please remember all of Autism needs to be investigated and developed and learned from not just the common version we have known for many years. In fact you have an obligation to investi-gate all of Autism not just what makes you happy.

For the benefit of my readers who might never get another or make another chance to experience Gay History I'm reprinting several highlights from the WEB site _QUEERS IN HISTORY._ I urge all my readers to view the web site as it spans centuries before christ up to the current times and such mainstream televi-sion programs as _Will and Grace_ and _Queer as Folk and Queer Eye for the Straight Guy._ History if not rewritten in a skewed manor is very informative and serves to enlighten. Thankfully in this day and age Gay is mostly accepted especially among the more educated populations and sadly many of those with an ax to grind might have some issues of their own to deal with. I am reminded of J. Edgar Hoover former Director of America's FBI a big bully who is most known for his anti Communist campaigns (and outing people) was gay himself. His listing appears below.

From the Website Queer History, a freely copied list, on the web at http// users.cybercity.dk/~dko12330/queerhis.htm. It includes links to the associated Outlist and the First Couples Page.

Ancient Egypt—Horus&Seth   Oraris&Seth

> Niankhknum&Khmumhotep(c.2450BCE) Two royal officials of the Old Kingdom, buried together in a single tomb. Although each was married with children, reliefs in their joint tomb show them kissing and embracing in a way usually reserved for married couples. *Prudish Egyptologists tend to claim that they're brothers, but there is no supporting textual evidence and the representations are all wrong for that. So these guys would be the first Queer couple!*

> King Neferkare PepyII& General Sisnet(c.2300BCE) *Alater story(c.1800BCE) has the King sneaking out of the palace at night to visit the general, who was his lover*

> Akhenaten c1350BCE &Smenkhkare

Late Antique Egypt—

> Arianus (late third/early fourth century CE) Roman official in Egypt known from literary and documentary sources. In several Coptic martyrdom's.

> *Taese& Tsansno (late 4th/early5th century) Two nuns published for lesbian activity(apparently with each other): from paper by T.Wilfong at recent APA meeting.

> Papapollo & P-hello (sixth century CE) *Known from the Manuscript of a love spell in which Paparpollo is trying to compel the love of P-hello (both men)*

Ancient Iraq—

> Gilgamesh&Enkindu

Ancient Greece—

> ? All Spartan Men
> All Cretan Men
> The Sacred band of Thebes {military regiment} 378-338 BCE

Mythical persons included for interest's sake (Latin in parentheses)

> Zeus (Jupiter)& Ganymede (sometimes "Catamitus"—origin of word 'catamite—Latin)
> Poseidon (Neptune) &Pelops
> Apollo& Admettus
> Hyacinthus (see below) & Cyparissus
> Dionysius (Bacchus) and Prosymnus
> *Artemis (Diana)&Callisto
> *Athena(Minervia)&Pallas
> Pan Achilles&Patroclus
> Hercules (Hercules)& Hylas&Iolaus
> Thesus&Pirithous
> Damon& Pythias
> Orestes&Pylades
> Thyris&Corydon
> Laius (father of Oedippus)& Chrysippus
> Narcissus&Ameinias
> Orpheus
> Hyacinth (above), Thamyris, Zephyrus& Boreas

Transgendered mythical figures

> Hermaphrodites
> Cybele
> Tiresias
> Caenis/Caeneus (same person)

Generals, Kings and Leaders

> Antyus 4th century BCE
> Aristides d.c.486BCE
> DionysiiusII of Syracuse r.367-353 BCE
> Alexander of Pherae 369-358 BCE
> Periander of Ambracia
> Solon c.600BCE

Hipparchus of Athens late 6th c BCE
Aristogetion& Harmodius (supposed founders of Athenian democracy)
Alcibiades 450?–404 BCE
Themistocles c524–c459BCE & Stesilaoes of Keos
Demosthenes 384–322BCE
Archelaus of Mecedonia r.413-and Crateeas (one killed the other)
Phillip II of Macedon 359–336BCE
Alexander the Great 356–323BCE & Hephasteion

Poets & Writers

Sappho c 610–c580 BCE
Alceausc c620–c580BCE
Meleagerc c 100 BCE
Theocitus early 3rd c. BCE
Thegnis of Megara early 6th century BCE
Aeschines c390–322 BCE
Philostratus 2nd 3rd century BCE
Ibycus th C BCE
Anacreon 582?–485? BCE
Pindar of Thebes 518–c.446BCE& Thrsyblus
Theoxenus & Rfinus
Euripides 485–406 BCE
Sophocles 496–406BCE
Agathon c.425BCE
Strato
AchilliesTatius, Greek novelist wrote "Leucippe&Cleitophon"
Lucian of Samosata 115–180

Intellectuals

Phraedrus 5th century BCE
Phaedo of Elis 5th century BCE
Socrates 469?–399BCE
Plato 427?–347 BCE
Zeno of Citium c333–262 BCE, founder of Stoicism.
Shrysippus c280–207BCE, Stoic Philosopher
Apollpdrous c140BCE, Stoic Philosopher

Ancient Rome

Kings, Emperors, Generals, and Political Leaders

Lucius Quinctius Flamininus c180BC
Sulla c.138–78BCE And Metrobius
Catiline d.62 BCE
Julius Caesar 100?–44BCE {Every women's husband, every man's wife}
& Nicomedes, King of Bithynia
Mark Anthony c82–30BCE
Cicero 100–43 BCE& Octavain/Augustus b.63–r27BCE
Tiberius r.14–37
Caligula r.37–41 (Inter Alia)
Nero r.54–68
Vespasian r.69–76
Titus r.79–81
Domatian r.81–96
Hadrian r76–138 &Antinous d.130
Marcus Aurelius r.121–180
Elagabalaus r.218–222, declared one of his male lovers to be his husband

Poets, Intellectuals

Catullus 84–54BCE
Horace 65–8BCE
Martial 40–103/4
Virgil 70–190BCE
Tibellus 55–19BCE and Marathus
Ovid 43BCE–17
Juvenal c2nd C CE
Petronius d.65, wrote the Satyricon
Plautus 250–184 BCE
Seneca 4BCE–65

Ancient biblical Figures

? The men of Sodom c.1800 BCE disputed story in Gen19
?*Ruth c. 1100 BCE and Naomi
David 1035?–960? BCE and Jhonathan I sam19 or IISam26
Daniel the Prophet c.650BCE, (eunuch')

The Three Young Men c.650BCE {eunuchs}
? St. John the Evangelist 1st C CE
? St Paul 1st C CE and Timothy

Medieval Europe and Islam

*St. Anastasia the Patrician
*St Anna/Euphemiamos
*St Apollinaria/Dortheos
*St Athansia of Antioch
*St Eugenia/Eugnios
*St Hilaria/Engnios
*St Marina/Marinos
*St Marina (2)
*St Matrons/Babylas
*St Pelagia/Pelagios
*St Theodora/Theodorus
*St Euphrosyne/Smargdus
*St Papula of Gaul
*St. Thekla
*St Hildegonde of Neuss near Cologne

All of the above women dressed and lived as men usually monks.

*St.Uncumber (a bearded woman saint)
St Sergius & St. Bacchus
St.Perpetua and St.Felicity
St. Sebastian
St.Augustine of Hippo 4th C
St Aelred of Rievaulx early 12th C
St Inseam of BCE late 11th C
St Paulinus of Nola 4th C and Ausonius

Other Religious Figures

? The Cathars[aka bougres]
St Alcuin 9th century
Gottschalk
Hrbanus Maurus
John Bishop of Orleans (aka "flora")
John of Salisbury 1115 or (1120)–1180 & and Pope Hadrain IV

Marbod of Rennes
Ralph, Archbishop of tours 12th C
Venantius Fortunauis
Walafrid Strabo & Luitger
Baudri of Bourgeuil 1046–1130
Pope Benedict XI 1020–1055
? Pope Boniface VIII b.c. 1235–r.1294–1303 charged with "sodomy"
by Philip IV of France
Pope Julius II
Pope Sixtus IV 1471–1484 contemporary diarist claims he made his
barber cardnial, because
he was his lover's son.
Pope Julius III1487–1555 and the Prevostino
Giovanni della Casa 1503–1557, prelate and writer and fonder of the
Papal index
Sister Benedetta Carlini of Pescia c.1619

Byzantium

Nicephorus I r.802–811
Michael III r.842–867 and Basil I r.867–
Constantine VIII r.1025–1028
ConstantineIX Monomachus r.1042–1055
"Monastery of the Aguares" specifically for the eunuchs the most well
known sexual minority.

Iberia

Moshe ibn Ezra (poet)   Ibn Barzel (poet)
Ibn Sahl (poet)   Ibn al-Farra (poet)
Ibn Sheshet (poet)   Abraham ibnEzra (poet)

Judah Halevi
King al-Mutamid of Seville 11th C and Ibn Ammar (poet)
?King John II of Castille r.1406–1454 and Alevaro de Luna?
King Henery IV of Castille 1425 r.1454–1474, (called "la puta" by the
people) and Gergario Maran~on
Antonio Perez 1535–1611 Philip II of Spain's secretary of state
King Affonso VI of Portugal r.1656–1683
Francisco Correa Netto c1664 {Sacristan of Cathedral of Silves and

erotic letter writer} And Manuel Viegas (guitarst) &Juan Pacheco, Marquess of Vilena

Italy

Political Leaders

Emperor FredrickII d.1250
King Conradin of Sicily 1252–1268 and Frederick of Baden
Benedetto Varchi Venetian Ambassador at Rome
Filefilo
Politian
Bracciolini
Duke Ferdiniand II of Tuscany 18th C
Duke Cosimo III of Tuscany 18th C
Gian Gastone
Prince Ferdinand
Cardinal Francesceo Maria

Figures in the Arts

Donatello 1386–1466
Pietro Aretino 1492–1556
Pomponia Leto 1428–1498
?Nicclo Machiavelli 1469–1572
Andrea Poliziano 1454–1494
Leonardo da Vinci 1452–1519
Raphael 1483–1520
Michelangelo Buonarroti 1475–1564 and Tommaso Cavaleri
Giovanni Antonio bazzi "ill sodoma" 1477–1549
Giambattista Marino 1569–1625 (writer)
Caravggio 1573–1610
Benevenuto Cellini 1500–1571
Tasso 16 C (writer)
Niccolo Capasso 17 C (Neapolitan Dialect poet)
Antonio Rocco mid 17C, wrote "Alcibiade Fanciullo a Scuola" 1652 (gay love story)

FRANCE

Political Leaders

King Philip II Augustis r.1179–1223 & Richard the Lionheart (see Britain)

King Charles IX r.1550–1574

King Henery III r.1574 and his mignons Mougeron, Eperon, and Joyeuse

Count of Anjou late 16 C (HenryIII's brother) &Bussy D'Amboise

King Louis XIII b. 1601–r–1610–1643 and Baradas & Marquis de Cing Mars and Saint-Simon

? Cardinal Mazarin 1602–1661

Others

? The Templars, religious military order, suppressed early 14 C

? Jacques le Mollay, leader of Templars at dissolution

Gilles du Rais 1404–1440, mass murderer

*St Joan of Arc c. 1412–1431 and *La Rousse and *Catharine de la Rochelle

Moliere1621–1673 and Michel Baron

Theophile de Viau 1590–1626 (poet)

Jacques Valle des Barreaux 1599–1673 (poet)

Denys Sauginde Saint Pavin 1595–1670 (poet)

Francious de Metel, Abbe de Boisrobert1592–1662 poet and founder of the French Academy

BRITAIN

Kings, Queens and Political Leaders

King William II Rufus 1056?–1100

Robert Duke of Normandy late 11th C

William Aethling (son of henery I early 12th C

? King Henry II b.1133 r.1154–1189 and St Thomas a Becket c.1118–1170, Very doubtful but the basis of a play by Anouilh

King Richard I the Lionhearted b.1157 r.1189–1199 and Philip II Augustus, and Saladin, and Blondel and Raife de Clermon

William Longchamp, bishop of Ely (justiciar of Richard II) early 13th C

King Edward the II 1284–1327 and Piers Gaveston and then Hugh Dispenser

? King Richard the II b.1367 r.1387–1399
Sir Walter Raleigh 1554–1618
King James I&VI 1566 r. (Scotland) 1567 r. (England) 1603–1625 and
Lord Hay and Robert Carr and George Villiers, Earl of Buckingham

Others

Nicholas Udel 1505–1556
Christopher Marloew 1564–1593 Authored the First list of Gay People
? William Shakespeare 1546–1616
Richard Bar(n)field 1574–1627
Lord Southhampton 16C
Earl of Oxford 16 C
Charles Arundel 16 C
Francis Bacon 1561–1626, (scientist)
Anthony Bacon 1558–1601

Elsewhere in Europe

Hoeldrin
Erasmus of Rotterdam 1466–4536 {Humanist} And Servatius Roger
and William Blount, Lord Mountjoy
Theodore Beza 1519–1606 (Calvin's successor at Geneva) and Aude-
bert
Jerome Duquesony 1602–1645 (Flemish Sculptor)

Islam

Abu Nawas d.810 Arabian Poet
Caliph Muhammad al-Amin 9th Cent CE
Saladin 12th century (ruler of Egypt and Syria)
Omar Khayyam (persian Poet wrote "Rubbayat")
Ibn al-Farid 1182–1235 (poet)
Ibn Khaldun (historian)
Mehmet II al Fatih 1430–1481 Conqueror of Constantinople 1453

MODERN EUROPE post 1700

Britain, Political Leaders

King William III b.1650 r.1689–1702
*Queen Anne 1665–1714 and Sarah Churchill, Duchess of Mar-

loborugh
Lord Hervey 1696–1733 {George II's Prime Minister} and Stephen Fox
Horace Walpole 1717–1797 first Prime Minister
John Wilkes 1725–1797 radical politician
Alexander Carlylr late 18th c Scottish churchman
Charles Townshend late 18th C politician
Sir Hector McDonald1853–1903 General
Viscount Esher 1857–1930 General
Early Beauchamp 1872–1938 Leader of the Liberal party194–24–1931
General Charles Gordon 1833–1885
Horatio Herbert Kitchener 1850–1916
Robert Baden Powell 1857–1941 founder of the Boy Scouts
Roger Casement 1864–1916
*Christabel Pankhurst
Tom Driberg MP {Baron Bradwell} 1905–197?
Duke of Kent brother of King George V
Jeremy Thorpe Liberal party Leader (alive?)
Maueen Colquhoun MP
Lord Louis Mountbatten Admirial and Viceroy of India 1900–1971
Lord Avon Minister in Margert Thacher's 1st Administration

Poets, Writers

*Lady Mary Wortly Montagu and *Anne Wortley and *Honora Sneyd
Thomas Gray 1716–1771 and poet Norton Nichols
Mark Akenside 1744–1770 Poet and Jeremiah Dyson 1722–1776
Horace Mann 1701–1786
John Chute 1701–1776
William Beckford 1759–1844 and William Courtney
William Viscount Courtney 1773–1833 (? Same as above)
*Mary Wollstonecraft 1759–1797 and Fanny Blood
Lord (George Gordon) Byron 1788–1824 &lord Clare,& John
Eddleston & Nicolo Giraud
Richard Heber 1773–1833 book collector
Horatio Brown 1856–1926, writer on Vinice
Cardinal John Henry Newman 1801–1890 writer and Catholic convert.
One of my first coming out Experiences was at the Columbus Ohio Newman Center Gay men's support group. A number of Larger Campuses have a

Newman Center.
Alfred Lord Tennyson 1809–1892 poet
Gerard Manley Hopkins 1844–1899 poet and Jesuit
Edward Carpenter 1844–1929 social reformer
John Addington Symonds 1840–1893
Walter Pater 1839–1894 art critic
Norman Douglas 1868–1952 writer
Algernon Swinbourne 1837–1909 poet
AC Benson EF Benson Robert Hugh Benson writer (?) all the same
James Barrie 1860–1937 wrote Peter Pan
Frederick Rolfe, Baron Covo 1860–1913 writer
Lawrence Housman 1865–1959 social reformer
Oscar Wilde 1894–1900 Writer and Wit And Lord Alfred Douglas
Andre Raffalovich (dilletante) & Cannon John gray Poet and preist
*Vera Britten writer and *Winnifred Holtby writer
Roden Noell 1834–1894 minor poet
Marquis of Lorne 1845–1914
James Elro Fletcher 1884–1915 port, & J.D. Brazeley 1885–1970 classical Scholar-Greek vases
James Agate 1879–1947
Hugh Walpole 1884–1941 writer
DH Lawrence1885–1930 writer
TE Lawernce (of Arabia) 1888–1935 Writer and Soldier & Salim Ahmed (Dahoum) (see Dedication of "Seven Pillars")
? Robert Graves writer
W.H. Auden 1907–1973 poet
Duncan Grant
E.M. Foster 1879–1970 writer
Denton Welch writer
Evelyn Waugh 1903–1966 writer
Saki (H.e.Munro) 1870–1916 Short Story Writer
Wilfred Owen 1893–1918 poet
Siegfred Sassoon 1886–1967 poet
Harlod Nicolson 1886–1982 writer and politician
Somerset Maughham 1874–1964 writer & Gerald Haxton
*Radclyffe Hall, wrote "The Well of Loneliness" & Una Troubrige
* Virginia Woolf 1882–1941 writer and feminist & Vita Sackville-West {gardner}

* Violet Trefusis
* Mary Renault 1905–1983 writer & Julie Mullard
Joe Orton 1933–1967 writer & Keith Halliwell d.1967
A.E. Housman 1859–1936 poet & Moses Jackson
Forrest Read 1875–1947 writer
Stephen Tennant
Harlod Action Antoine in Waugh's Brideshead Revisited
Robin Maugham writer
Christopher Isherwood 1904–1986 writer and Don Bachardy Artist
Noel Coward 1899–1973 writer and actor
J.R. Ackerly writer
Lytton Strachey 1880–1932 biographer
James Kirkup poet
Robert Croft-Cooke writer
Lawrence Olivier 1907–198? And Danny Kaye see N America

Musical Figures

Authur Sullivian 1842–1900 composer
Benjamin Britten 1913–1976 composer and Peter Pears tenor
Ivor Nevello 1893–1951 composer
Brian Epstein 1934–1967 manger & John Lennon singer
Of course some day SIR Elton John will be added to this list.

Others

Andrew Baxter 1688–1750 Scottish Dutch moralist
* Marianne Woods early 19th C And Jane Pirie, Edinburgh School teachers
The Ladies of Llangollen
C.J. Vaughn c.1850 Head master at Harrow
Sir Richard Burton 1821–1890 19th century explorer and writer
Sir Edmund Blackhorse 1873–1944, sinologist
Charles Ricketts 1866–1931 artist and Charles Shannon 1863–1937 artists
Henry Tuke 1859–1929 artist
Goldsworthy Dichinson 1867–1932, Academic-Kings College
Ronald Gower 1845–1916 architect
John Maynard Keynes 1883–1946 economist

*Florance Nightingale 1820–1910
William John Bankes d. 1855 Dorset MP and early Egyptologist

Alan Turing breaker of the Nazi Enigma code *Rich's hero Autistic?*

Guy Burgess Spy for USSR subject of film "Another Country" & Tolya
Francis Bacon d1993 painter
Aleister Crowley (Witch)
Derek Jarman 1942–1994 Filmmaker
* Dolly Wilde 1899–1941 Oscar's niece, A "wit"
Lord Montagu Subject of Famous trial in 1950's
Cecil Beaton photographer
Ludwig Wittgenstein 1889–1951 Philosopher
? All students at Eaton since its foundation!
? All students at Harrow 1456–1917,1923–1969!

GERMANY/AUSTRIA

Political Leaders

Frederick II the Great of Prussia 1712–1786 and Hans von Katte
Prince Henry of Prussia 1762–1802 (suggested as King of America)
King Ludwig II of Bavaria 1845–1886
Fredrich Krupp 1854–1902, industrialist
Kaiser Wilhelm II 1859–1941 (r 1883–1918) &Prince Philippe zu Eulenberg 1847–1921
Colonel Alfred Redi early 20 C (Austrain double agent)
Ernst Roehm, (Nazi Leader)
Rathenau (German foreign minister at Versailles 1919)
Wilfed Israel 1899–1944 opponent of Nazis

Cultural Figures

?Ludwig von Beethoven 1770–1827 composer and nephew? Karl
?Franz Schubert 1797–1828 composer
J.J.Winklelmann 1717–1768 art historian
Count August von Platten 1796–1853, poet &Cardenio/Hoffman
Wilhelm Jansen 1866–1943 gay activist
Stefan George 1868–1933 poet & Maximilien Konberger
Karl Ulrichs 1825–1895, first person in modern history to acknowledge his homosexuality
Karol Kertbeny (=Benkert) Hungarian, invented the word homosexual.

Magnus Hirschfeld 1868–1935 sexologist
Baron Hermann von Teschenberg late 19C Transvestite and Gay Rights leader
Bendict Fiedlaender gay rights advocate
*Anna Ruehling late 19C lesbian feminist
*Rosa von Branschweig late 19C writer and activist
*Gabriele Reuter writer
*Marie-Madeleine Baroness von Puttkamer, poet
*Elizabeth Dauthendey, writer
*E Krause, writer
George Polck, Gay Rights advocate
Dr. ernest Burchard, Gay Rights Advocate
Otto Spengler, Gay Rights Advocate
? Rainer Maria Rilike 1875–1927, Poet &Frida Kahlo
Alexander von Humboldt explorer and scientist
*Rosa von Praunheim film maker
Thomas Mann 1875–1955 writer
Rainer Werner Fassbinder, film maker

Other

Ludwig le Gros &Martin Schultze, both executed 1704
*Catharina Margaretha Linck &Catharina Margaretha Muehhahn c. 1721
Baron Ludwig Christian Gunther von Appel c 1730

France

Political Life

Philippe, Duc de Orleans d.1701 brother of Louis XIV
Eugene of Savoy
Louis, Prince of Conde
*Madame Anne-Louise Germaine du Stael 1766–1817
*Marie Antoinette 1755–1793
Violet-le-Duc
Duc de Nevers
Eugene Sue
? Maximilien Robespierre1785–1794 &? Saint Just
Duc Claude de Villiars
? Napoleon I Bonaparte 1769–1821 Emp. 1804–1815

Jean Jacques Regis de Cambaceres 1753–1824, designed Code Napoleon

King Louis XVIII

Daniel Guerin social activist

Cultural Figures

?Voltaire 1694–1778

Paul Henri Dietrich thiry, Baron d' Holbach 1723–1789 philospher,

Francois Timoleon de choisy Abbe de Choisy 1644–1724

Marquis de sade 1740–1814

Marquis de Custine 1790–1857, writer on Russia

Theodore Gericault 1791–1824 painter

*Georges Sand 1804–1876

Comte Robert de Montesquiou 1855–1921 poet

Paul Verlaine 1844–1896 poet & Arthur Rimbaud 1854–1891

Camille Saint-Saens 1835–1921 composer

Jean Cocteau 1889–1963 writer& Raymond Radiguet

Jean Genet 1910–1986 theif and writer

*Colette 1873–1954 writer

Andre Gide 1869–1951 writer & Athman

*Anais Nin 1903–1977 writer and diarist

Henri de Montherlant 1896–1971 writer

Marcel Proust 1871–1922 writer &Reynaldo Hahn1874–1947

*Renee Vivien 1877–1909

*Rosa Bonheur 1822–1899 & Nathalia Micas

Max Jacob 1876–1944 poet

Francois Poulenc 1899–1963 composer & Pierre Bernac

*Marguerite Yourcenar 1903–1987, writer, first woman in French Academy

Roland Barthes Lit critic

Russia

Tasr AlexanderI 1777–1825

Nikolia Przhevalsky 1840–1888 explorer

Peter Tchaikosky 1840–1893 composer (Merry Chr stmas!)

Vaslav Nijinsky 1890–1950 dancer & Filosof & Sergei Diaghelev 1872–1929

Sergei Rachmaninov 1873–1943 composer

Mikhaill Kuzmin 1875–1936 poet
G.V. Chicherin 1872–1936
Rudolph Nuryev 1938–1993 dancer

Elsewhere in Europe

*Queen Christina of Sweden 1626–1689 & Ebba Sparre
? Giacomo Casanova 1725 1789 (!)
Ali Pasha c.1744–1822 Alabanian Political Leader
? Hans Christian Anderson Denmark, writer
Jillis Bruggeman, Netherlands, subject of famous sodomy case 1803
Pontus Winker 1837–1888, Swedish Philosopher
Cernuda Spain
Frederico garcia Lorca 1898–1936 Spain, writer
Constantine Cavafy 1863–1933, Greece poet, & Anastssaides
Peir Paol Pasolini 1922–1975 Italy, Film maker
*Florbela Spanca Portugal, poet Baron von Gloeden
*Dona Catalina de Erauso
*Isak Dinesen 1885–1962 Denmark Poet writer
Erik Thorsell 1899–1980 Sedwish Iron Worker wrote autobiography
on his Gay Life
Karol Szymanowski 1883–1937 Polish composer
*? Anne Frank 1929–1945 Netherlands diarist
Dag Hammarskjold 1905–1962 sewden UN Sec General
Pope Paul VI 1897–1976

North America

Pre Conquest

I-coo-coo-a early 19th c Souix (Lakota) berdache
Sahaykwisa C1850–1895 Mohave

Political Leaders

?Edward Hyde Lord Cornbury 1661–1724 Governor of New York
1702–1708
? President George Washington 1732–1799 & Alexander Hamiliton
(speculative)
Alexander Hamiliton 1755–1804 & John Laurens 1754–1782, com-

pared them selves to
Damn and Piths

? President James Buchanan 1791–1868 & Sen. William Rufus de Vane
King 1786–1853
* Susan B. Anthony 1830–1906
Bayard Rustin 1910–1987, organizer 1963 March on Washington
Walter Jenkins 1918–1985
J.Edgar Hoover 1895–1972, head of FBI & Clyde Tolson 1900–1975
& Terry Dolan
Roy Cohn 1927–1986 McCarthyite Lawyer
• Eleanor Roosevelt 1884–1962 First lady and Us Ambassador to UN
Woman of the year & Lorena Hickok, journalist

Writers

Henry James 1843–1916
Herman Melvile 1819–1891 & Marnoo & Nathenial Hawthorne
1804–1864
Henry David Thoreau 1817–1862& Edmund Sewall
*Emily Dickinson 1830–1886 &Sue Gilbert
Ralph Waldo Emerson 1803–1882&Martin Gay
Horatio Alger 1834–1899
*Jane Bowles 1917–1973
John Horne Burns, Wrote The Gallery
Thorton Wilder 1897–1975
*SaraTeasdale 1884–1933 & Margret Conklin
Tennesse Williams 1911–1983
*Jane Chambers 1937–1983
Angelina Weld Grimke 1880–1958
Paul Goodman 1911–1972
* Maragret Fuller 1823–1850
*Lorain Hansbury 1930–1965
*Gertude Stein 1864–1946 & Alice B. Toklas
*Charlotte Cushman and Emma Stebbins
*Mercedes de Acosta
* Ivy Compton-Burnett
* Elizbeath Bowen
* Alice James
*Sarah Orne Jewett

*Carson Mc Cullers
*Liane de Pougy
*Margaret Anderson
*Dorothy Baker
Truman Capote 1924–1984
* May Sarton
* Maureen Duffy
*Edith Hamiliton
Walt Whitman 1919–1982
James Baldwin 1924–1987
*Willa Cather 1876–1947 & Isabella McClung
John Cheever 1912–1982
Hart Crane 1899–1932
Langston Hughes 1902–1967
Alan Locke 1886–1954 & Richard Bruce Nugent
*Audre Lorde 1934–199?
*Edna St. Vincent Millay 1892–1950
Colin Higgins 1941–1988
Robert Ferro
Howard Sturgis 1855–1920
*Sylvia Beach 1887–1962 & Andrienne Monnier
Harry Beecher Ward 1813–1887
James Barr wrote Quarterfoil
Merle Miller 1919–1986
Alan Barnett
George Stambolian
Alan Bray
*Natalie Barney 1876–1972
*Romanie Brooks 1874–1970 & Djuna Barnes 1892–1982

Hollywood and Broadway

*Tallulah Bankhead,
James Dean 1931–1955
* Greta Garbo 1905–198?
Errol Flynn 1909–1959
Cary Grant
James Whale 1896–1957
Rock Hudson 1925–1985

Charles Laughton 1899–1962
Sal Mineo
George Cukor 1899–1983
Charles Ludlam
Danny Kaye
Bill Sherwood, directed Parting Glances
Luchino Visconti 1906–1976
Kenneth Anger
Montgomery Clift 1920–1966
Rudolph Valentino 1895–1926
Richard Burton
Parker Tyler
* Alla Nazimova Nancy Reagan's godmother
Raymond Burr d.1993 Perry Mason

Music

Divine, Drag Diva Died the night before debut on TV's Married With Children
Ma Rainey 1886–1939
Bessie Smith 1898?–1937 singer
Liberace d.1987 Pianist
Alberta Hunter 1895–1984
Leonard Bernstein 1918–199? Composer
Araon Copeland 1900–199? Composer
Stephen Foster 1826–1864
Samuel Barber 1910–1981 composer &Gain Carlo Menotti
*Janis Joplin pop singer
Cole Porter 1892–1964 songwriter
Sylvester disco diva

This list and the other lists on the website including The Outlist (Living People) could fill volumes. I left out of this list Africa, Latin America Asia, Japan and Australia. I encourage you visit the website and experience the whole thing for yourself. I included this part of the list to prove the point that being Gay, BI sexual Lesbian and Transgendered is as natural as being left handed. Gay Folks as you can see have been around forever and many have been great leaders. Only in the stereotypes are we made out differently. Today the Symbol of Gay Pride the world over is the Rainbow flag, and it can be seen every place on earth. What other flag of a nation or a religion has truly universal appeal? Perhaps the Coca-Cola wave sign is the only other thing on earth with universal recognition. Gay it seems was here long before religion was invented when man learned to read and write and I suspect it will be here long after time has proven religion to be worthless. You know it could be just simply be Mothers Natures attempt at population control?

I am in no way suggesting that all Autistic people are Gay, Transgendered, BI sexual etc. But those of us that are and the wear-with-all to come out had a definite advantage growing up mainly, a premade social group. Gay Folks who were typically bashed in school from the "in" crowd (in earlier days) were generally welcomed in this group. What other MR/DD type of population gets accepted into any type of social group? That Acceptance and tolerance taught many of us the social graces we needed. For those of you that think this book is too gay, I remind you Gay made this book possible. Autism success as you have seen is indeed a hampered by many things. Changing a few variables in the experiment made a world of difference. This was like Queer Eye for the Straight Guy, the popular TV show in many respects. With out our gay social graces we would present totally different and might never have developed an Autism Interface for social things.

If you're in need of help with Gay Issues, P-Flag Parents and Friends of Lesbian and Gays has many chapters nationwide and their mission is help in coming out and support for all. Also many United Church of Christ churches are Gay Friendly as are the Universal Unitarians. Today one also finds pockets of Acceptance in the Methodist, Lutheran and other churches. By the way, Exodus an EX Gay Group is a big joke, and it success rate of converting Gays to straight is dismal and doesn't even consider the pain inflicted on it members.

13

Conclusion July 2003

Dear Reader's

The Autism Spectrum will never be the same again! All of the 'experts' that claim 'expert' status have just been set—back a few years—to a point and time before Rain Man, when Autism was pretty much a solved and workable condition. Perhaps, a time before 'anything was considered Autistic'. It would be ludicrous to throw all of modern Autism out the window on purpose as many dedicated, honest and sincere people have really given there all to the cause. However with the "new" but yet tried and true information presented here disproves lots of the Post Rain Man Autism theory. Even what Autism is needs to be questioned. Some of it needs tossed out the window and we need to build and blend the rest of it in to a workable Autism like we once enjoyed. It might be TOO late we have to over come Rain Man's image that has even filtered into the likes of the television shows like ER and Law and Order and mainstream publications like Good Housekeeping Magazine. Stereotypically the Autistic is portrayed as some off center unsociable type of genius. PLEASE/ER with out Pain Tolerance and a millinthrong of lost doctors and nurses is just a lie.

Autism and its older typically undiagnosed (gay perhaps) people the world over, prove time and again that Autism is not MR/DD unless it is treated as such. Latin is a better description of Autism and it is obvious those of us that figured out the Latin of Autism have made it. Autism the modern version doesn't like to look for it lost legions at all, let alone in Gay circles, it is bad for funding. It also refuses to search the lower edges of civilization to look for those of us that made it and are typically just getting by living on the streets or in a rooming house. We think naturally with Picture Thought we adapted normal thought like you use and most of us live normal lives and drive. Since we have been there and done that, our Autism Answers—shoptalk—if you will when we talk among ourselves is far different and more 'correct' than modern Autism would ever expect. If only

Post Rain Man Autism non-profits will accept this invitation to talk with us and discover us perhaps they might do everyone in the spectrum a great service.

However I'd literally be quite shocked to see a one of them give up their guns admit a few mistakes and get on with the VITAL business of treating Autism correctly. Autism is pretty much an established fact these days, and in reality it was never understood to start with. I wonder that IF Rain Man hadn't made so many good points Autism would have been different, almost unknown and yes boring to the point only those effected would be involved in the spectrum. It would have never made buzzword status and thus the 'boring' Autism that it really is would be better understood by now. Perhaps, the kids that really are Autistic and not feeling the injuries that afflict them and those termed as low functioning not responding to sing-a-longs and efforts at eye contact would not be so bad off. Even today IF picture thought were taught like I suggest in this book and presented to everyone Autistic, those with that natural ability and thought process would be most thankful for having their learning style presented to them. Those in the spectrum not likely to Picture Think would not be out too much and if this doesn't do anything for them. We could then send them to other classes teaching traditional methods.

Once this reaches publication and gains a wide spread reputation—I get the bees buzzing around the hive—I can see all kinds of possible trouble from current Autism. Perhaps, they are just too far entrenched in their ruts by now to even admit to us. Of course, in their eye were all high functioning and thus not autistic? But let me assure you to be high functioning we started out at low functioning.

I wonder if a smear campaign would not be in order? The Political Action Committees and the dollars at RISK may make it worth while to smear each and everyone of the worlds High-functioning People into the dust. If they discredit us to throw off world off the point, and then hopefully we will die before to much longer as many of us are older than the Rain Man era person: then they can go on blissfully ignorant. It is their idea of every one wins. The researchers have good jobs and reputations that are unchallenged by those of us figuring out Autism for ourselves and the Autistic lives life in a group home. What could be better?

Sometimes the world's best ideas are lost due to politics and normal thinking form Traditional Thinkers. I can think of the Lustron Homes of the 1950's, Metal prefab homes that were the perfect answer to America's housing shortage in that era. The idea was killed as few politicians hated the idea. Washington made a scandal of the idea and of course years later the 2500 or Lustron homes made are still standing and those responsible for the stink have all been jailed for lying under oath. In another case of normal thinking, A man in the same era by the name of Demming (A Bell Labs engineer) presented to the powers at be his idea on factories, workers and workmanship and doing all in a way that everyone won. He was' Laughed Out of town" He took his message elsewhere and today the best and most trusted names in QUALITY all bear his input. Perhaps, Toyotas are American cars after all.

Then one can't help but worry that they will give us lip service, "like us long enough to glean some of our secrets" and do another Rain Man farce on those in the spectrum. The Traditional Thinkers they are will feel empowered with our secrets and think for the love of themselves that can duplicate our experience and turn it into the 'Perfect Autism School '. They didn't even get the point with Temple's Thinking in Pictures (obviously) so it will not be a great shock to see them ruin this as well. Granted if they copy us it will be a better Autism learning experience than anything currently offered, but, it will still miss some of the finer points, the points that need to accounted for, in order for their Autism education to work, like ours did. Add to the mix the education and social issues, psychology and the Medical Science 'Fiction' aspect that they have basically never experienced and it spells Autism that needs to be fully investigated and accounted for. Sadly, I predict lots of people diagnosed Autistic will be found, not to be Autistic and that alone will be reason enough to hate us and wipe us out.

If I don't get too badly damaged and beat up with this experience I encourage my counterparts world wide to write their own acccunts of Autism. It is our only chance to save future generation's form Rain Man's Fate. I strongly urge my readers to stop supporting the Current Autism Establishment with their hard earned money, as they have already done you a great dis service by not studding and elevating all of Autism's Obvious Answers that are there for the taking? No Thinking or research required. IF our experience was ever accounted for/the face of Autism would be wildly different and might look like some of the stuff Temple Grandin, presented. Overall success and failure in Autism is indeed a FINE line.

Socially we might have been the only 'population' accepted into a social group, growing up? I remember the tormenting the normal kids did with the special populations in our school, and now realize had I been straight and Autistic, no one would have cared enough to make me their friend. I would have been the big loser with out that positive experience. The straight undiagnosed Autistic I speak with today all seem to do Autism well, and think in pictures etc., But you can tell they missed out on the charm school offered by being Lesbian, Gay, Transgendered or BI Sexual. In fact when all is said and done Autism will have learned its brightest points and most important facts from the Transgenederd in our population. These dear people whom I consider my friends have done Autism with a twist that even the Gay Population never had to endure. That Extra Experience will prove invaluable to Autism.

I really hate to reinvent the wheel again, and would love to be accepted as a group into the current Autism societies but that might be an Impossible Dream. The Profits form this book will be donated to Autism as I cannot make a profit off of some other person's misfortune. I assure you I will be really careful and try not to be duped (excellent statement for someone autistic to make) into a false sense of being accepted to get our money. In fact if none of the Big Non-profits currently in Autism will be honest sincere and forthcoming, we will start our own Autism non-profit and hopefully will not have to spend a lot of our time or resources fighting the current establishment. One of the FIRST goals of this effort whether as part of the current autism team or on our own will be Autism text books—the "Mc Guffy Readers" of Autism—The next goal will be a School totally set up and run by Autistics to teach Autistics. We might not be perfect, and for sure it will be a learning experience for everyone. We have to a better job than anyone else ever could, we have already figured out Picture Thought. No other "Expert" can claim that privilege.

This book has been 9 years in the making now and it had been presented to nearly everyone in the Autism spectrum and no one including the Autism Society of America or Dr. Rimland responded to it. A BIG Autism publisher was presented with this book (an early version) in stages. They loved the book and could not wait to get a hold of it. My last E-mail from them after they finally seen the whole book, Gay included, was rather short and nasty. "We no longer publish personal stories of autistic people." Well I have seen their list in recent years and they do, but I suspect they are straight folks. Prior to the introduction of Gay, It was a great book and one of their employees called it Temple Grandin type of stuff. I had purposely sent the initial pages of the book to them in such a way just the technical stuff was presented; Gay was finally presented when it came time to expose the whole book. I went from saint to sinner pretty quick. This is why this was published outside the Autism spectrum.

For those suffering from unknown injuries, 'The Barbarians" of modern medicine have some catching up to do. Please do your level best to stay healthy. Chances are you do not feel enough internal pain to tell you or the doctors something is wrong. My best doctor understanding my whole medical history tells me he would put me in a coma for 6 weeks after an operation to keep me from tearing myself to pieces again. I am horrified of anything internal being done such as a scope type procedure. I could be punctured and pinched somehow and never feel it. I have walked into the Doctors office three days after an operation and never felt a thing when I should have been on pain pills and crutches! Basically the deeper in something is the less of it we feel. I have been to the heath dept. for just in time life saving treatments (IV meds) when I was so sick I was losing weight quickly and had a rash from head to toe. Our best guess was an intestine might be injured and leaking which is logical considering my physical injuries. I have no insurance so medical tests and "proper" care was not available. The Health Dept. was doing its best to keep me going by trading for drugs I needed and pulling all kinds of strings.

A kind word to the Psychologists reading this, I appreciate your degrees and experience and the efforts you put forth on behalf of your profession. I do wonder about some of you although, perhaps you prescribe too many pills in an effort to keep folks under control so that you might not get a phone call ruining your weekend? I really feel sorry for some of the families and parents you serve. I can't fault you however, your are all doing approved practice. Sadly, Autism among other things in this world is only in the infancy of understanding so mistakes will be made. Please, keep in mind my Picture Thought explanations in mind as you go through your professional lives, they might prove to hold lots of clues to Autism as well as the human mind in general. I bet this is one of the first times this whole idea of a different thought process has ever been explained and for sure you didn't get it in your college courses.

To the Parents living with this on a daily basis, you are on your own as you well know. Perhaps, the Label of Autism is just too big of a deal for your friends, family and neighbors to deal with. You are indeed doing your best, and doing what your being told and giving the drugs that are being prescribed. That just proves how little is known of Autism. I suspect my Father and Mother would tell you (they were ignorant of Autism and drugs in that era) to impose strict discipline in your household, keep your house quiet and peaceful and identify splinter skills and take them to the limits. Eventually that knowledge will filter into the real world and connections can be made. They gave up on eye contact and social things possibly realizing I was not 'wired that way' and years later they discovered that stuff kind of developed on its own. Today Dad knows when I am thinking in pictures by the lack of quality eye contact and even waits for the thought to be converted and spoken before going on.

Finally, one last disclaimer, I have never met Temple Grandin other than for a few seconds. We have never talked in person or otherwise. I know her from her work and the various items written about her and of course, from her Fresh Air program interview. Her wonderful work sets the stage for this book and tells the world of our Picture Thought and different state of being. I used this writing to expand upon her work, and I hope someone some day will be able to the same do with mine.

I offer my apologies to those that think I might have slighted them, in this writing, slander, bad manors, getting even were never the intent but discovery was. I tried and tried to be heard and seen and recognized in official channels and was just ignored. I suspect the book would be totally different if the powers at be, hadn't been so obstinate but at least I am not beholden to anyone in the Autism spectrum. My views looking out and not in would mesh well anyway. By the way, I love the movie Rain Man and it is indeed a fine movie, It might sound like I hate it but to clarify it, I hate the results of Rain Man, I'm sure it was never intended to derail Autism research in any way but, thanks to the modern world and the show biz aspect of our modern times—Autism had no choice but to be held hostage to the times. Don't forget our "Autistic" hero Alan Turing, Father of the Computer, he might be the world's most famous "Autistic" if he were given due credit for his work.

Sincerely, Rich Shull Ohio, Usa. July 31, 2003

Websites to consider

My website   http://hometown.aol.com/austicrich/page 1.html
For the latest news about this book and new links to Autistic groups set up between my high functioning counterparts and the rest of the world. Several groups are geared toward the normal person and the Autistic person. Several groups are dedicated the Transgendered among us and another group is between Gay folks and Autistic Gay folks.

Alan Turing—Father of the computer.   Http://www.turing.org.uk/turing

Queers in History—Http://users.cybercity.dk/~dko12530/queers.htm

Irlen's syndrome (visual disorder) I Think Irlens Syndrome might be Picture thoughts trying to form.
Http://www.readingandwriting.ab.ca/judypool/irlen#irlen

Bread for the World   www.bread.org

BURNING Man—A yearly event   www.burningman.com

Rich Shull

austicrich@aol.com

0-595-29298-4